healthy everyday

High Protein

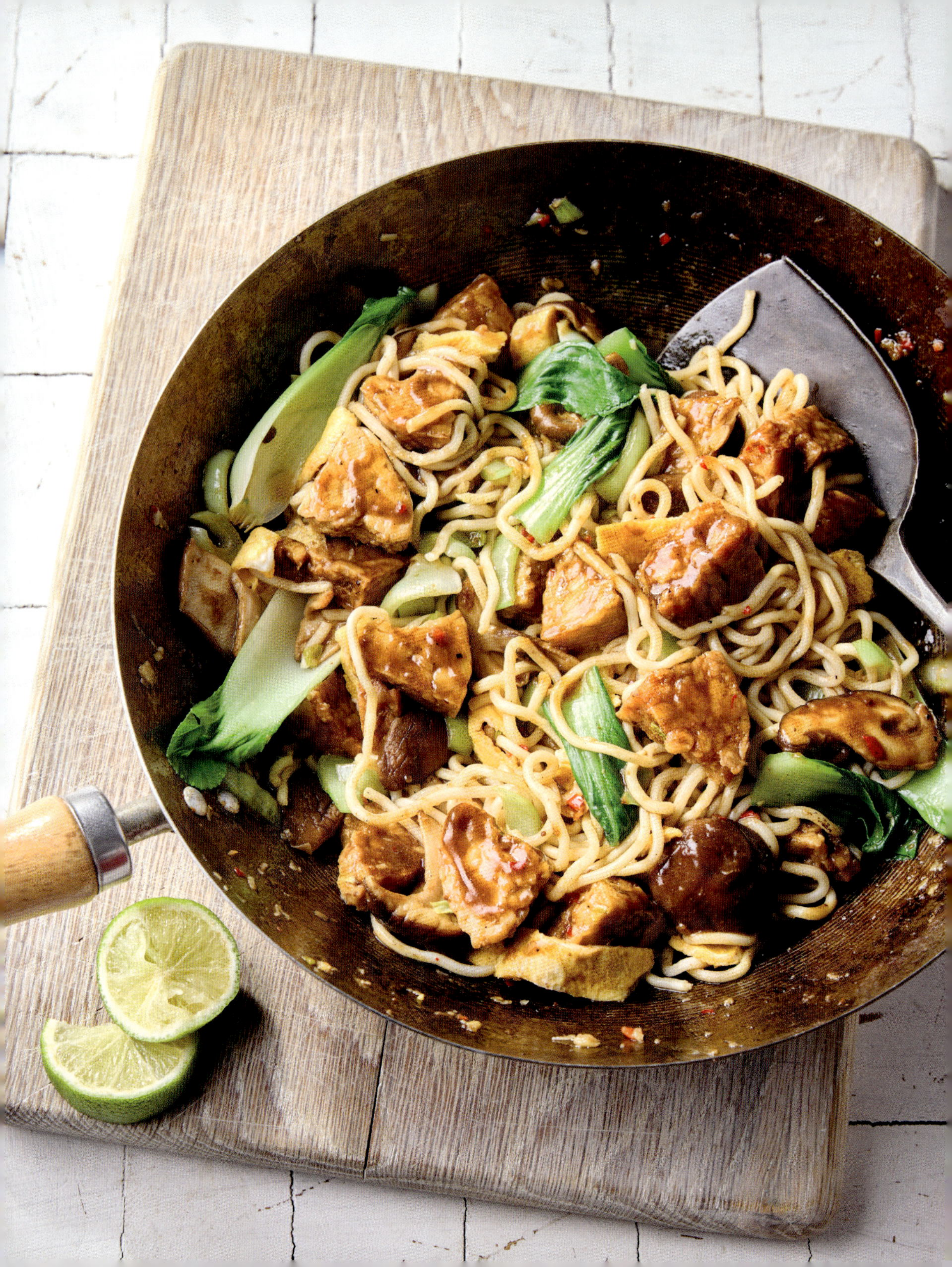

healthy everyday

High Protein

70 delicious recipes designed with nutrition in mind

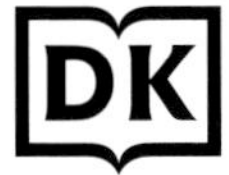

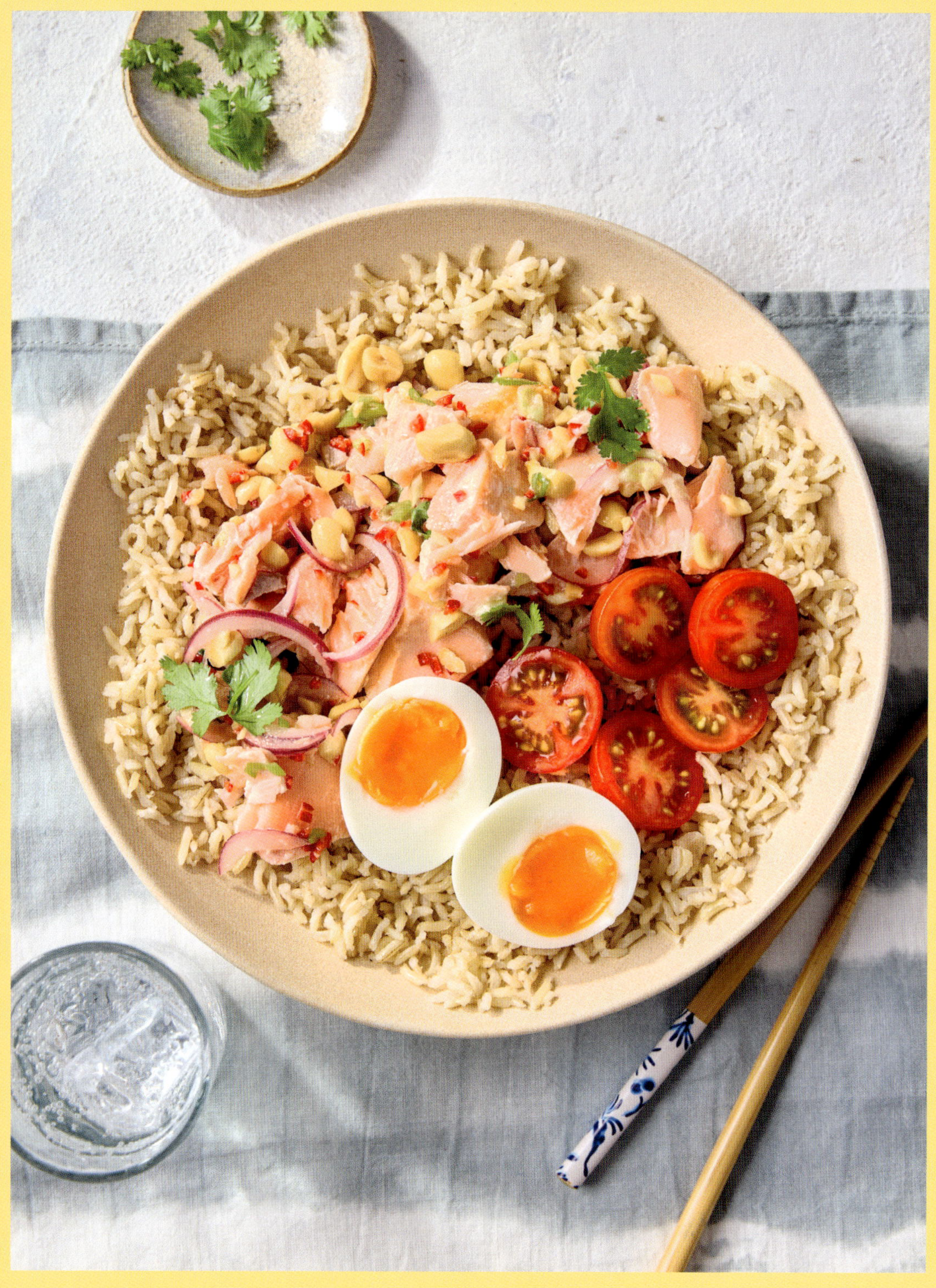

Introduction 06

Breakfast
18

Protein-packed Lunches
46

Midweek Dinners
68

Batch Cooking & Meal Prep
96

Air Fryer
128

Snacks & Sweets
148

Conversion Charts 170

Index 171

Introduction

We often find ourselves short on time, and healthy, balanced eating can quickly get pushed down the priority list. With simple techniques and a little planning, it can be easy to pull off quick, healthy, and balanced meals that are high in protein and keep you feeling fuller, for longer.

These recipes are not only high in protein, healthy, and balanced, but they cover every appetite and craving. Just because food is good for you it doesn't mean it can't taste good!

Why Protein Matters

Protein is a vital building block of life. Every cell in your body relies on protein to function and repair itself. When we eat protein, our bodies break it down into amino acids, the "building blocks" that fuel essential processes like tissue repair, immune defence, and even mood regulation.

There are 20 amino acids in the body, and nine of these are known as essential amino acids. Our bodies can't make them on their own, so we need to get them from food. That's why eating enough quality protein is so important for good health – especially during times of growth, aging, or hormonal change.

What Do We Mean by "High Protein"?

In this book, we define a high-protein meal as one that provides a meaningful amount of protein to support satiety, muscle and bone health, and metabolic function – amounts vary depending on the size of the meal you're having.

This framework reflects evidence-based guidelines for supporting energy levels, muscle maintenance, and appetite regulation – particularly helpful during midlife, for active lifestyles, or when you're focusing on recovery or strength-building.

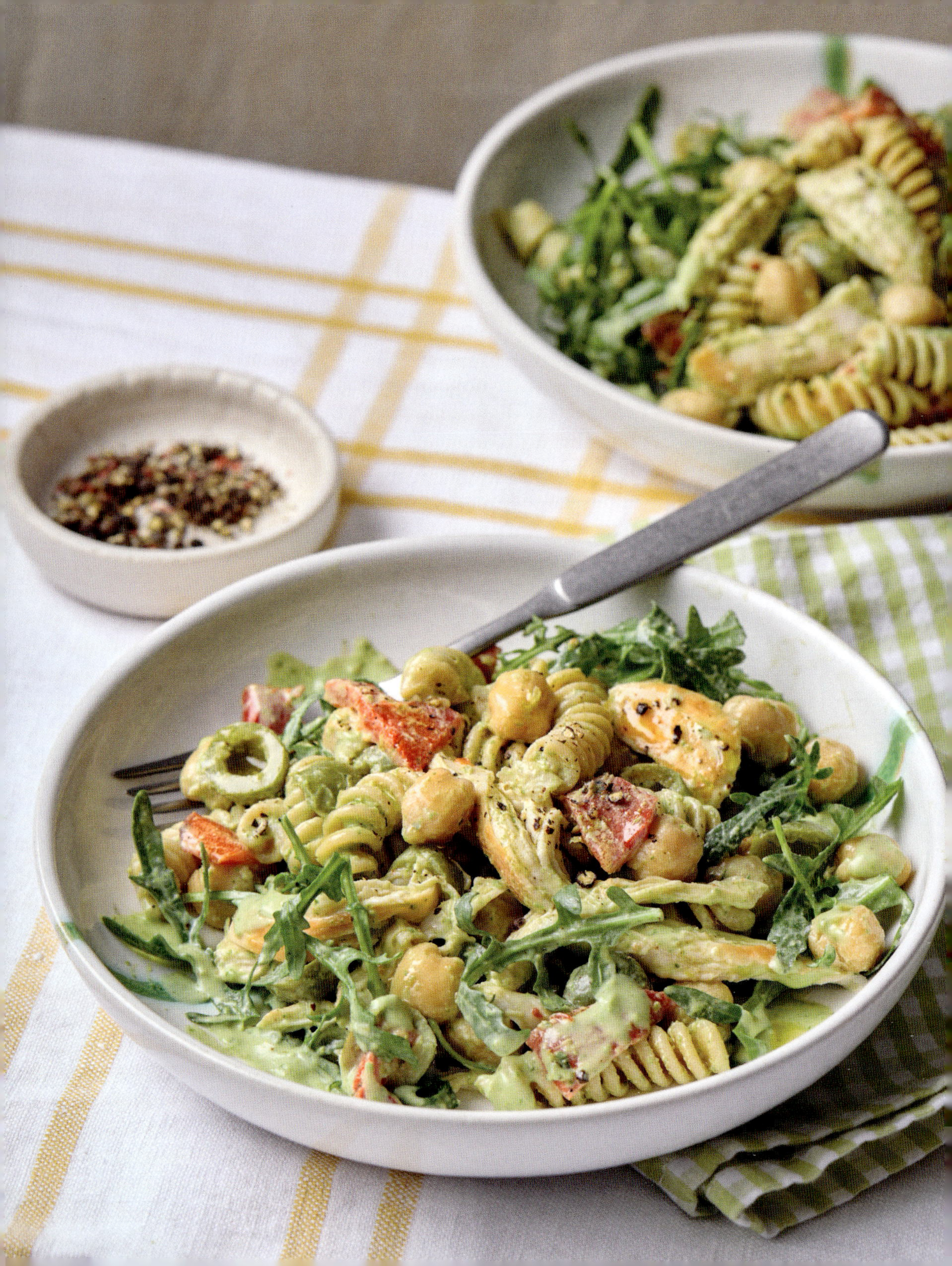

Where Do We Get Protein From?

Protein comes from a variety of sources, both animal- and plant-based:

Animal-based proteins include meat, poultry, fish, eggs, and dairy. These are considered complete proteins – they contain all nine essential amino acids. They're also rich in nutrients like vitamin B12, iron, and zinc.

Plant-based proteins come from beans, lentils, tofu, tempeh, quinoa, nuts, seeds, and wholegrains. Some are also complete, while others need to be paired with different plant foods across the day to ensure all essential amino acids are covered.

It's absolutely possible to eat a high-protein diet without meat, as long as you include a variety of plant-based sources. This variety is key, not just for meeting protein needs, but for getting a wide range of fibre, antioxidants, and micronutrients that support overall health.

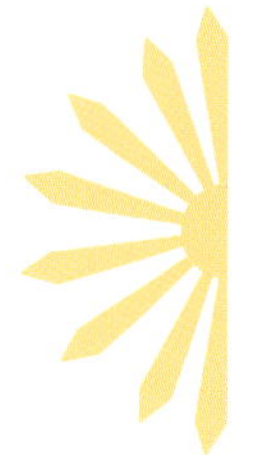

Variety is key, not just for meeting protein needs, but for getting a wide range of fibre, antioxidants, and micronutrients

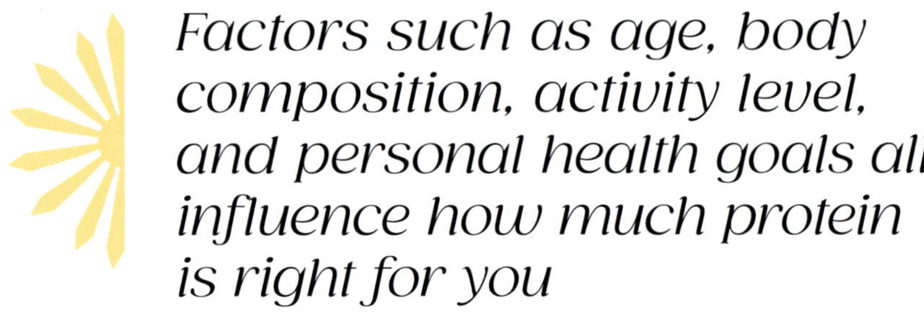

How Much Protein Do We Need?

The World Health Organization (WHO) recommends a minimum intake of 0.8g of protein per kilogram of body weight per day for adults. This is considered a baseline to prevent deficiency, rather than a target for optimal health.

Research suggests that higher intakes – around 1.2 to 1.6g of protein per kilogram of body weight per day – may be more beneficial for supporting muscle maintenance, appetite regulation, recovery, and overall wellbeing, particularly during periods of aging, increased activity, or physical stress. For example, someone weighing 70kg might benefit from 85–110g of protein per day, ideally spaced across meals.

That said, balance is key. Consistently very high protein intakes – especially above 2g per kilogram of body weight per day – may displace other important nutrients, if not carefully planned. A varied diet that includes adequate fibre, healthy fats, and a broad spectrum of vitamins and minerals remains essential for long-term health.

Factors such as age, body composition, activity level, and personal health goals all influence how much protein is right for you. This book offers flexible options to suit a variety of needs.

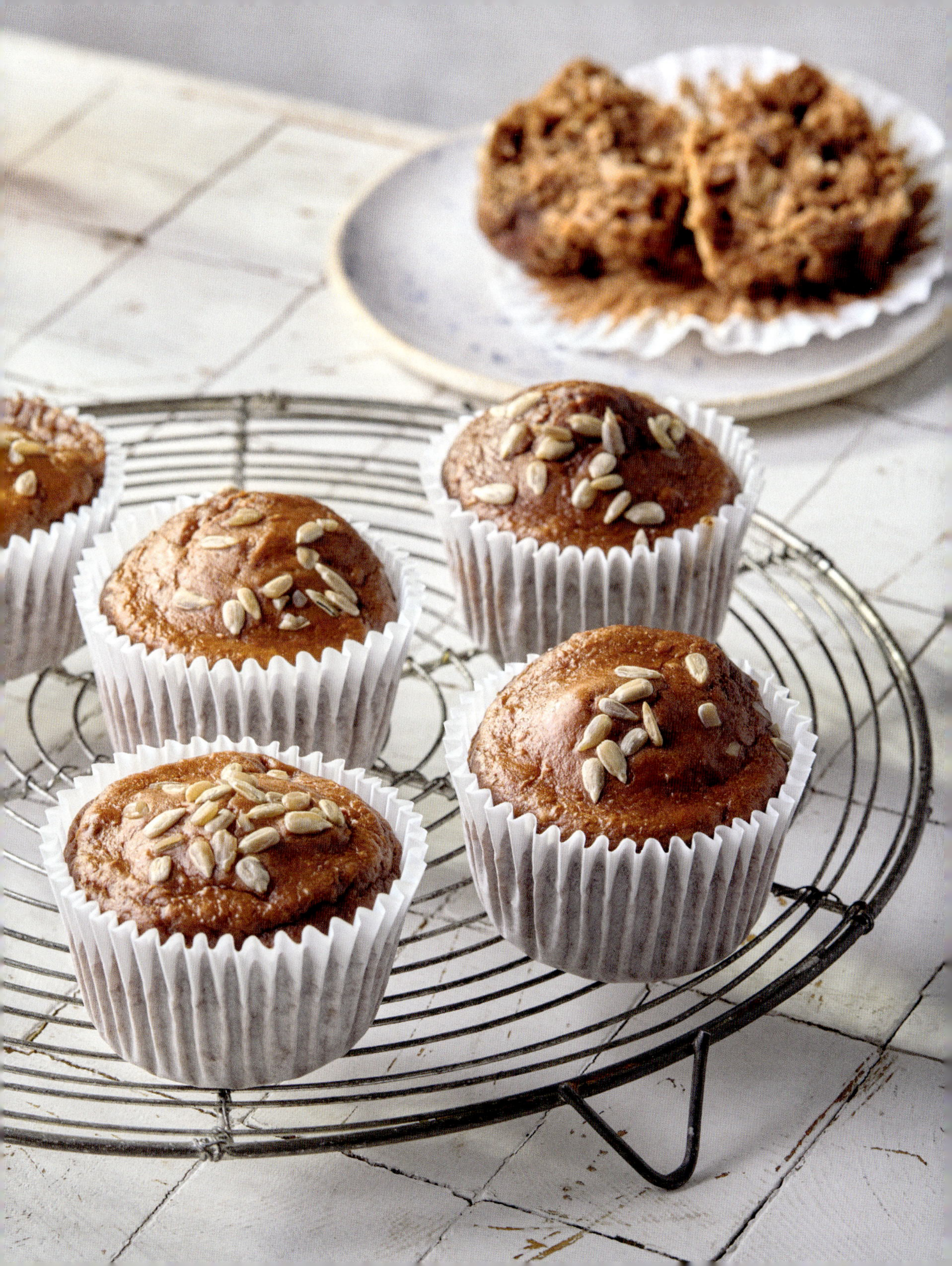

The Benefits of a Higher-protein Diet

Choosing to increase your protein intake – particularly from nutrient-rich, wholefood sources – can support a range of health goals, including:

Improved muscle maintenance and strength, especially during aging or the menopause

Healthy weight management, through increased satiety and metabolic support

Steadier energy throughout the day

Better appetite regulation and reduced cravings

Support for recovery after illness, injury, or intense activity

A higher-protein approach can be especially beneficial during periods of increased physical activity, recovery, or aging, when the risk of sarcopenia (age-related muscle loss) becomes more significant.

This is particularly relevant after the menopause, when hormonal changes can accelerate muscle loss and impact metabolism.

Prioritizing protein during these times can help support strength, energy, and long-term health, helping you feel more resilient, nourished, and able to meet the demands of everyday life.

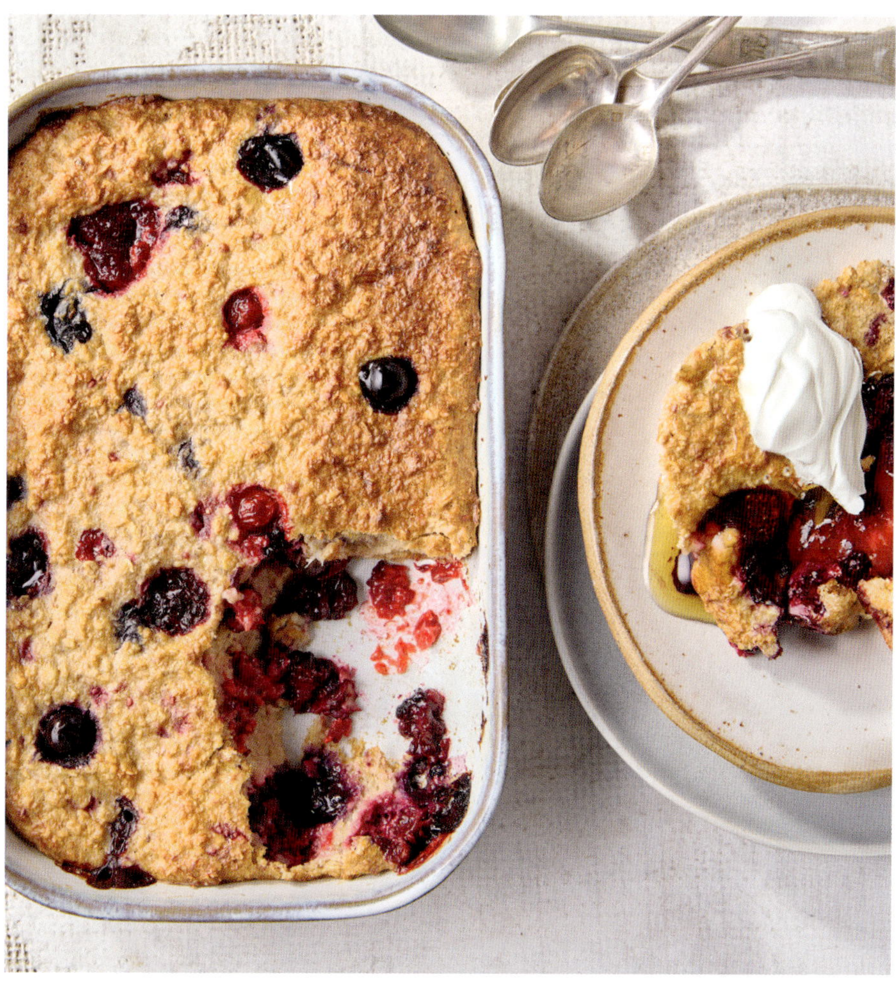

Tips and Tricks

Equipment

Making sure you have the right equipment to hand is important when following a high-protein diet. Here is a list of handy things to have in the kitchen:

* **Storage containers** are essential for batch cooking. Keeping your fridge or freezer stocked with pre-prepared meals is invaluable, for those moments when you don't have time to cook something from scratch.

* **Large pots and pans** will allow you to scale up recipes, so that you can prepare meals in advance.

* **A blender** will enable you to make fresh sauces, smoothies, and quick, healthy desserts.

* **A range of different-sized mixing bowls** will help you to prepare and organize meals, quickly and efficiently.

Hacks

There are a few tips and tricks that can make it effortless to add protein to your diet and ensure you're making nutritious meals often:

* **Meal planning** will ensure you are thinking about the amount of protein you are getting from each meal, and will guarantee that each meal contains some form of protein. It can also help you budget - doing one big shop at the beginning of the week and batch cooking will stop those impulse takeaways!

* **Filling the larder with high-protein staples** is essential. Canned beans, canned lentils, canned fish, and bags of lentil pasta are all great sources of protein, and when you haven't made it to the supermarket, whipping them out of the cupboard makes for a speedy way to rustle something up.

* **Adding nuts and seeds** when plating up a meal will give your meal an extra protein boost.

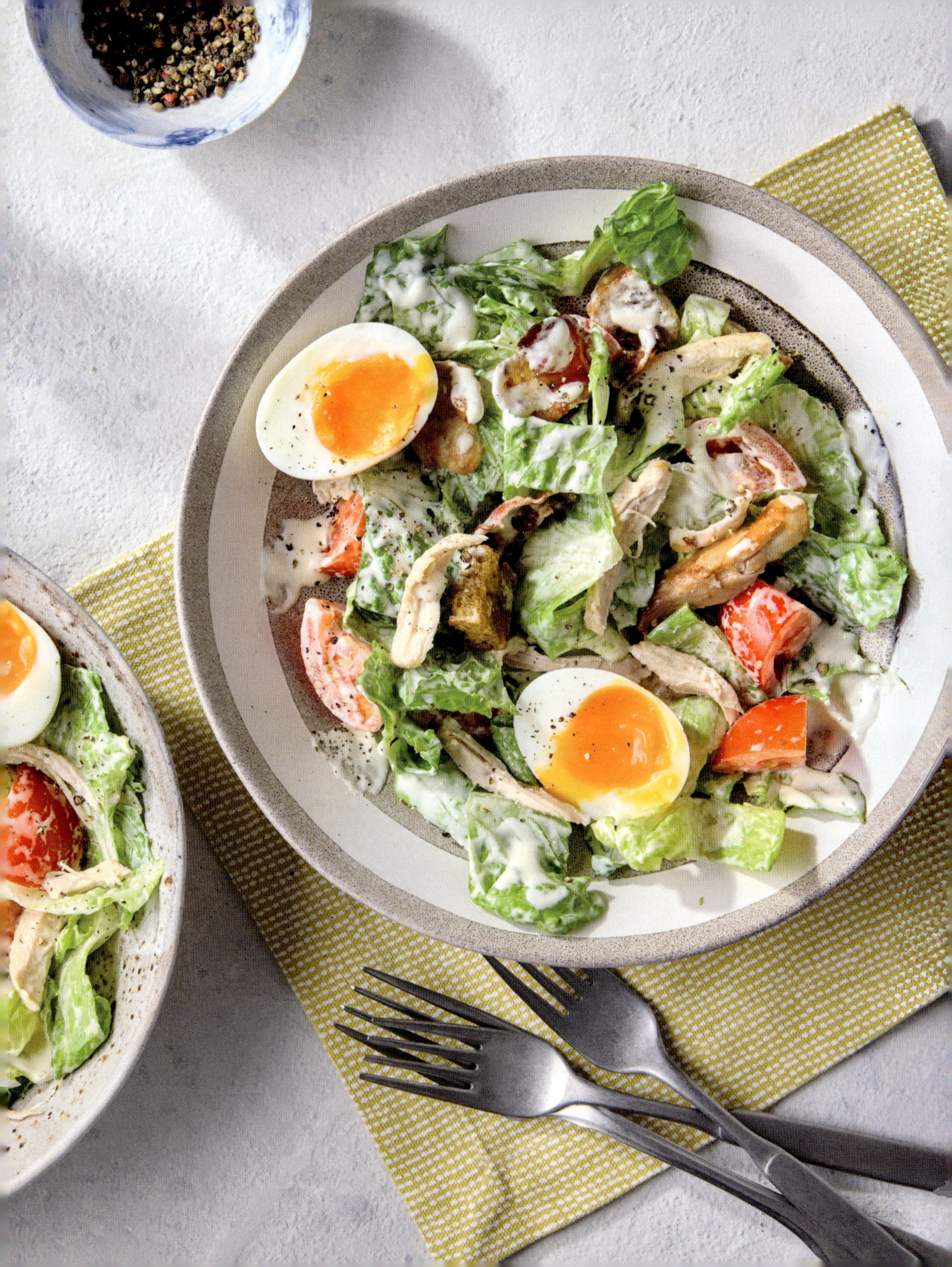

Meal Planner

Planning your meals for the week can be a great way to achieve your goals and pack protein into your meals. Use the grid below to make a note of your favourite recipes to stay on track.

	MONDAY	TUESDAY	WEDNESDAY
BREAKFAST	Masala Omelette (see p23) **Protein per serving: 24g**		
LUNCH	Tuscan-style Soup (see p54) **Protein per serving: 20g**		
DINNER	Chicken Tacos (see p137) **Protein per serving: 38g**		
SNACKS & SWEETS	Chocolate Mousse (see p169) **Protein per serving: 11g**		
DAILY PROTEIN COUNT	**Total protein: 93g**		

THURSDAY	FRIDAY	SATURDAY	SUNDAY

Breakfast

Starting the day with a high-protein breakfast is the most effective way to support sustained energy throughout the day and curb those mid-morning cravings. These recipes have been designed to help keep you feeling full and satisfied all the way through to lunchtime, using protein-dense ingredients like eggs, tofu, nuts, and seeds.

Smashed Peas on Toast

Protein per serving: 22g **Kcals per serving: 450**

Serves 2

Prep + cook time: 5 minutes

- 200g (1⅔ cup) frozen peas
- 1 tbsp extra virgin olive oil
- 2 slices of sourdough bread
- 150g (5¼oz) feta
- 4 radishes, thinly sliced
- pinch of chilli flakes
- grated zest and juice of 1 lemon
- salt and freshly ground black pepper

1 Fill and boil a kettle, then add the peas to a small saucepan. Once the kettle has boiled, fill the saucepan with boiling water and boil the peas on the hob for 1 minute.

2 Drain the peas, then add them to a bowl. Add the olive oil, season with salt and freshly ground black pepper, mash the peas with a fork, then set aside.

3 Toast the sourdough, then top with the smashed peas and crumble over the feta. Add the radishes, chilli flakes, and lemon zest, then squeeze over the lemon juice.

Swap It: Edamame beans would also work well here.

Peas are a lesser-known, but brilliant source of protein. When combined here with feta, they give this veggie option a real protein boost.

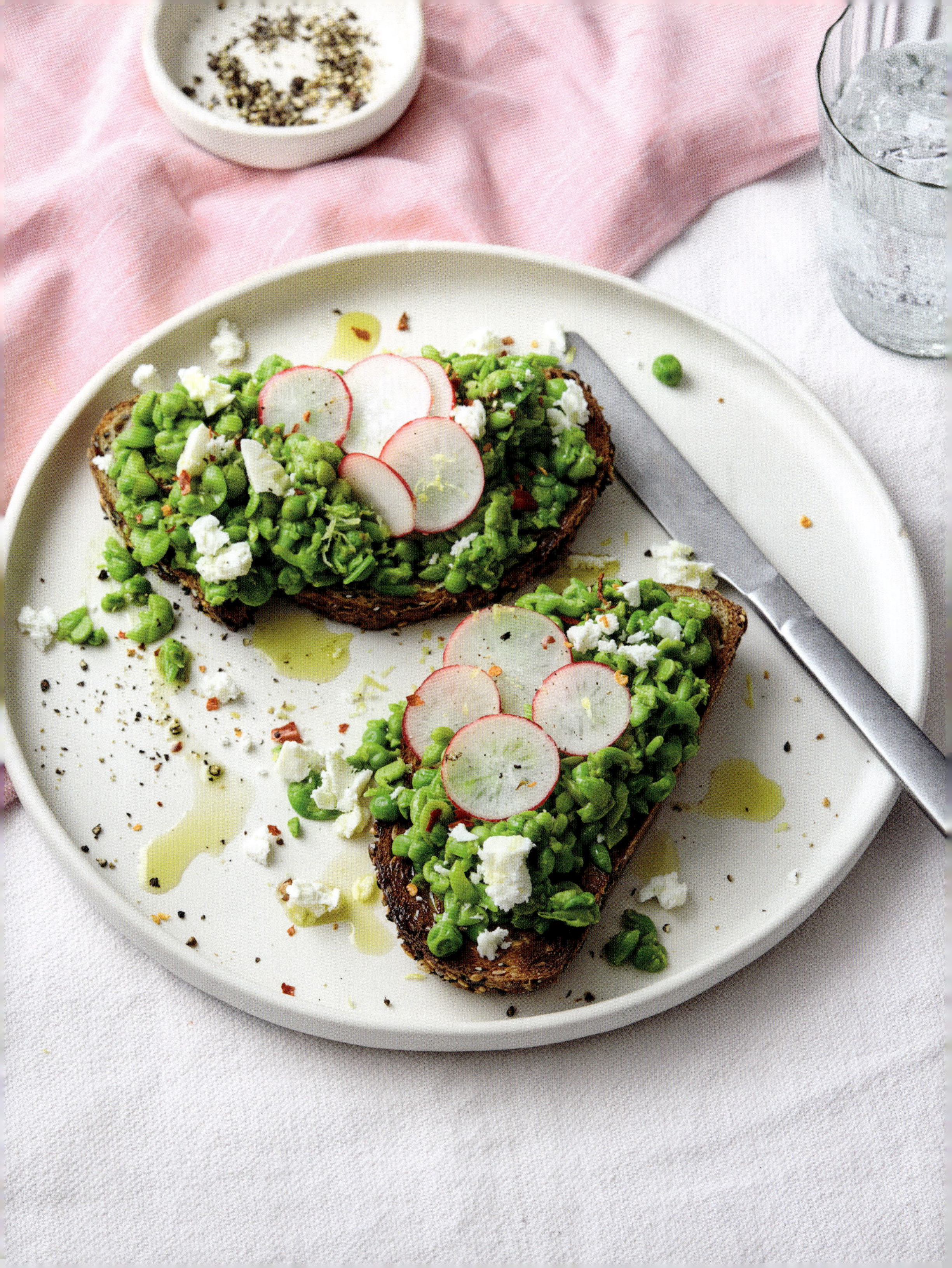

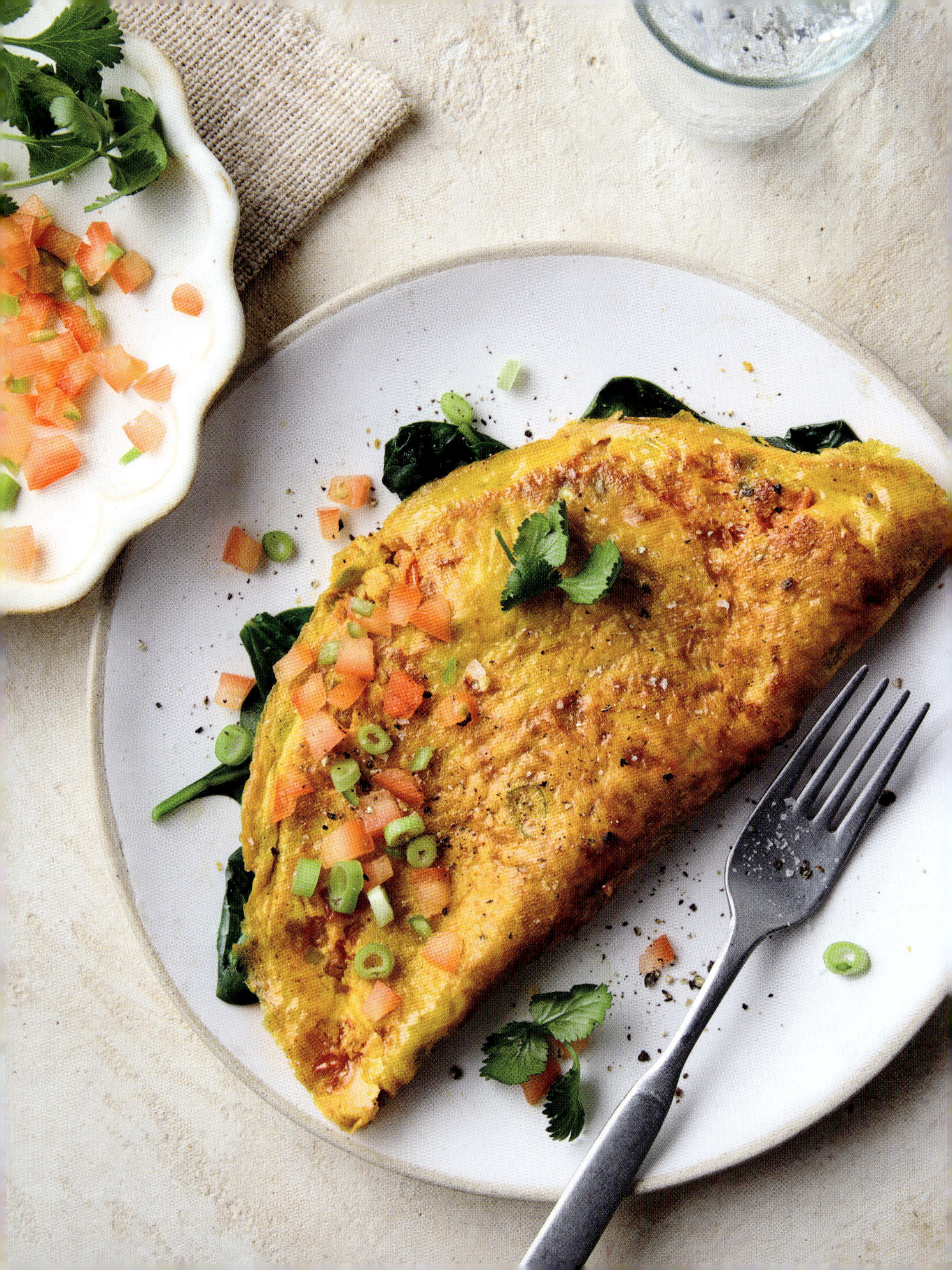

Masala Omelette

Protein per serving: 24g **Kcals per serving: 416**

Serves 2

Prep + cook time: 10 minutes

- 1 tbsp extra virgin olive oil
- 1 large tomato, deseeded and finely chopped
- 1 spring onion, finely chopped
- 1 tbsp lime pickle
- ½ green chilli, deseeded and finely chopped
- 4 large eggs
- 1 tbsp curry paste
- 50g (½ cup) grated Cheddar
- handful of spinach
- salt and freshly ground black pepper
- coriander leaves, to serve

1 Add the olive oil to a frying pan, then set over a medium heat. Set aside a pinch of the tomato and spring onion for serving, then add the rest to the pan with the lime pickle and green chilli. Cook for about 3 minutes until the vegetables have softened, then lower the heat.

2 Meanwhile, crack the eggs into a bowl, add the curry paste, then whisk well. Add in the Cheddar and spinach, along with a pinch of salt and freshly ground black pepper, and mix until combined.

3 Add the egg mix to the pan, then swirl the pan around, allowing the eggs to cover the surface of the pan. Let it cook for about 4 minutes until the egg is set.

4 Fold the omelette in half, then slide onto a plate and sprinkle over the coriander and reserved tomato and spring onion.

Tip: Leave out the lime pickle and curry paste to make this an equally tasty cheese and spinach omelette.

Eggs are nutritional powerhouses. As well as protein, they provide vitamins such as A, D, and B12 and minerals such as iron and choline.

Blueberry Pancakes

Protein per serving: 31g **Kcals per serving: 585**

Serves 2

Prep + cook time: 10 minutes

- 180g (generous ¾ cup) cottage cheese
- 3 large eggs
- 100ml (6½ tbsp) milk
- 120g (1⅓ cup) rolled oats
- 1 tsp baking powder
- 1 tsp ground cinnamon
- 1 tbsp maple syrup, plus extra to serve
- 1 tbsp vegetable oil
- 100g (3½oz) blueberries

1 To a blender add the cottage cheese, eggs, milk, oats, baking powder, cinnamon, and maple syrup. Blitz, then set aside for 5 minutes.

2 Add the vegetable oil to a frying pan over a low-medium heat. Add 70g (2½oz) blueberries to the pancake mix and stir through until combined. Add half a ladle per pancake to the pan, and fill with as many pancakes as you can, ensuring they do not touch. You may need to do this in batches. Flip after 2 minutes and cook for another minute until golden and cooked through.

3 To serve, top with the remaining blueberries and drizzle over some extra maple syrup.

Swap it: To make these savoury, leave out the blueberries and top with bacon.

The use of cottage cheese really boosts the protein content, as well as providing calcium for bone health.

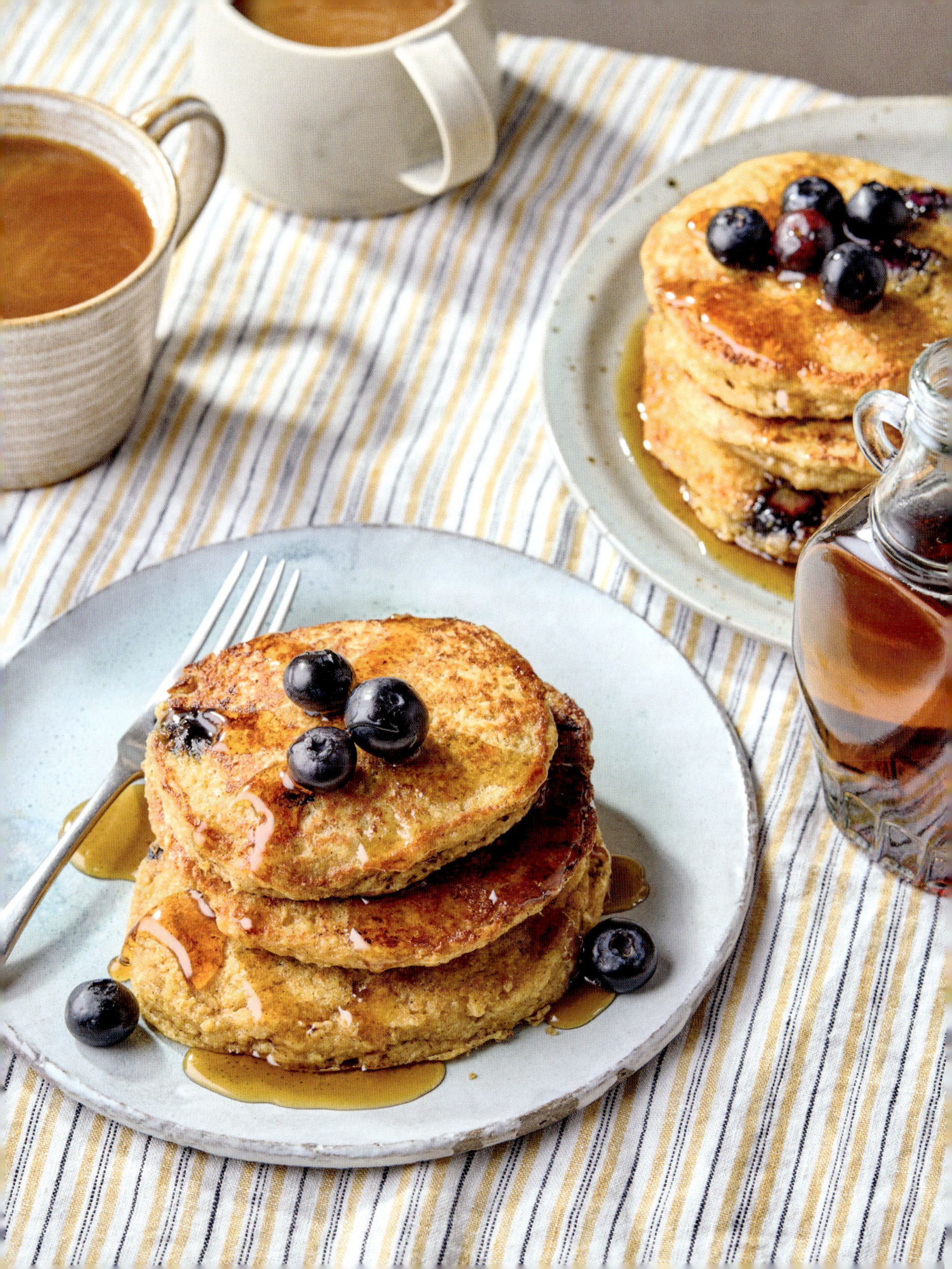

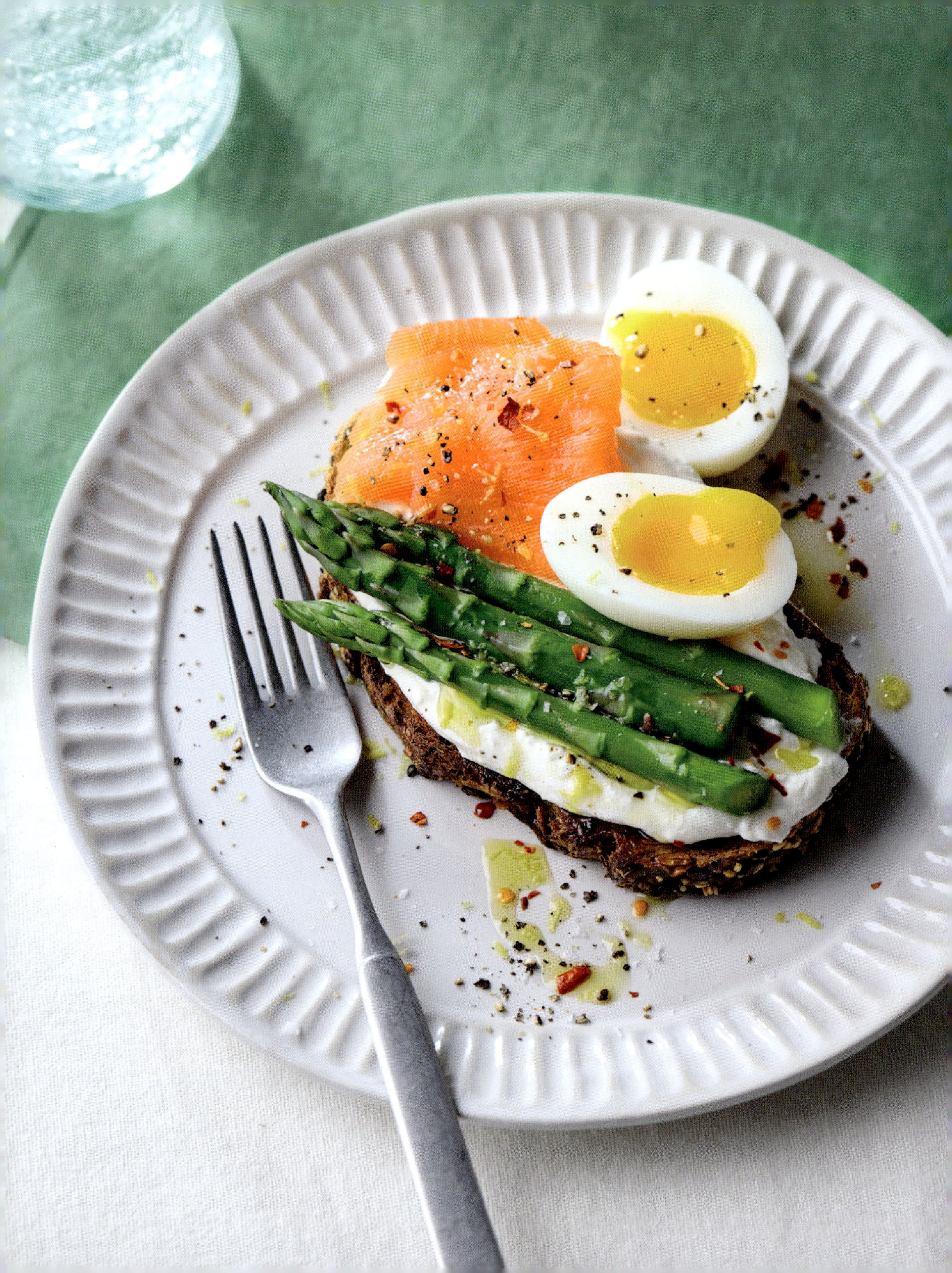

Smoked Salmon and Asparagus Toast

Protein per serving: 28g **Kcals per serving: 328**

Serves 2

Prep + cook time: 10 minutes

- 100g (scant ½ cup) cottage cheese
- 2 large eggs
- 100g (3½oz) asparagus, stalks trimmed
- 2 slices of seeded bread
- 100g (3½oz) smoked salmon
- grated zest of 1 lemon
- pinch of chilli flakes
- salt and freshly ground black pepper

1 Add the cottage cheese to a blender, then season with salt and freshly ground black pepper. Blitz until smooth, then set aside.

2 Fill a saucepan with water and bring to the boil. Once boiling, add the eggs to the pan and boil for 6 minutes. Remove the eggs and run under cold water to stop the cooking process. Set the eggs aside, and leave the water boiling.

3 Add the asparagus to the boiling water and cook for 1 minute until tender. Remove and set aside.

4 Meanwhile, toast the bread.

5 To assemble, spread the cottage cheese over the toast. Peel the eggs, cut them in half, and arrange on the toast. Top with the asparagus, salmon, lemon zest, chilli flakes, and a good crack of black pepper.

Swap it: To make this veggie, leave out the smoked salmon, and double up the quantity of cottage cheese for extra protein.

Smoked salmon is a source of protein and omega-3 fatty acids, which are essential for brain health.

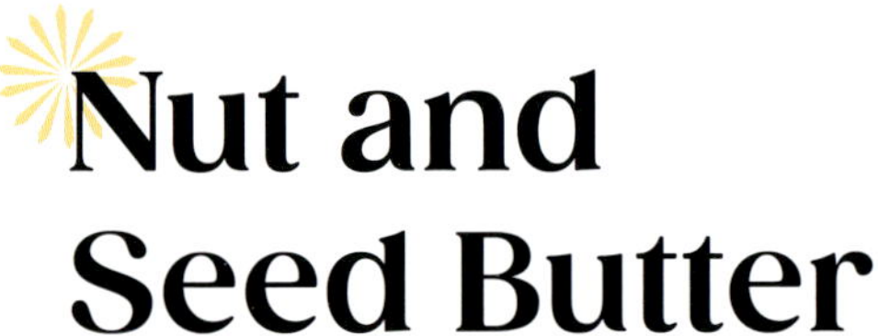

Nut and Seed Butter

Protein per serving: 17g **Kcals per serving: 461**

Serves 8

Prep + cook time: 20 minutes

500g (4 cups) cashews
100g (¾ cup) pumpkin seeds
30g (4 tbsp) flaxseeds

1 Preheat the oven to 180°C (160°C fan/ 350°F/Gas 4).

2 Add the cashew nuts and pumpkin seeds to a baking tray. Put the tray in the oven and cook for about 8 minutes until lightly golden.

3 Add the nuts, seeds, and flaxseeds to a blender and blitz for 10 minutes, scraping down the sides at regular intervals. It should look smooth and creamy and be a runny consistency.

4 Transfer to a sterilized jar and store for up to 1 month in the fridge.

Swap it: This is such a great way to use up leftover bags of nuts and seeds in your pantry. Swap in and out for whatever you may have. You could simply just use nuts here.

As well as protein and fibre, cashews provide magnesium and copper, which both play a role in energy production.

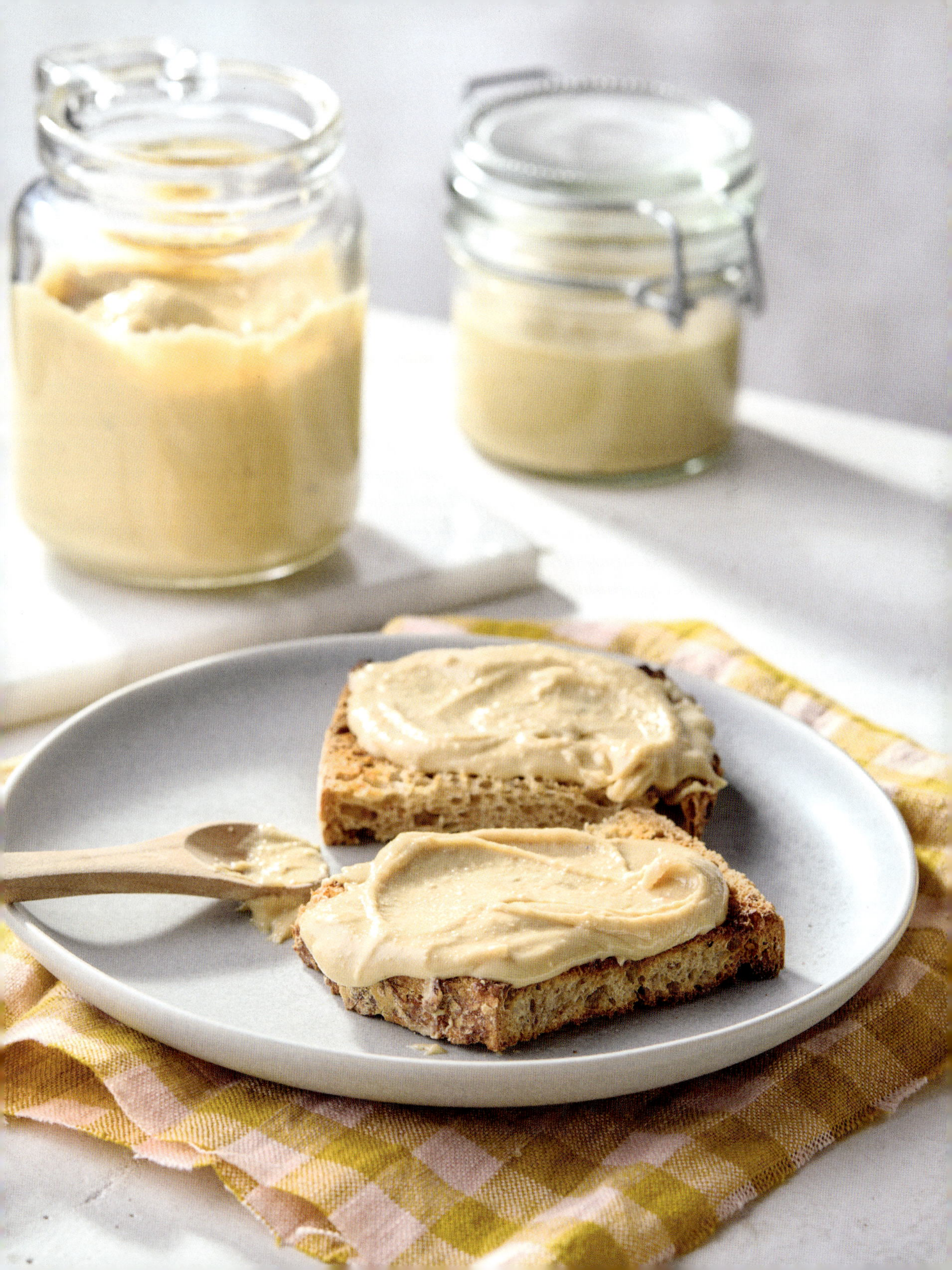

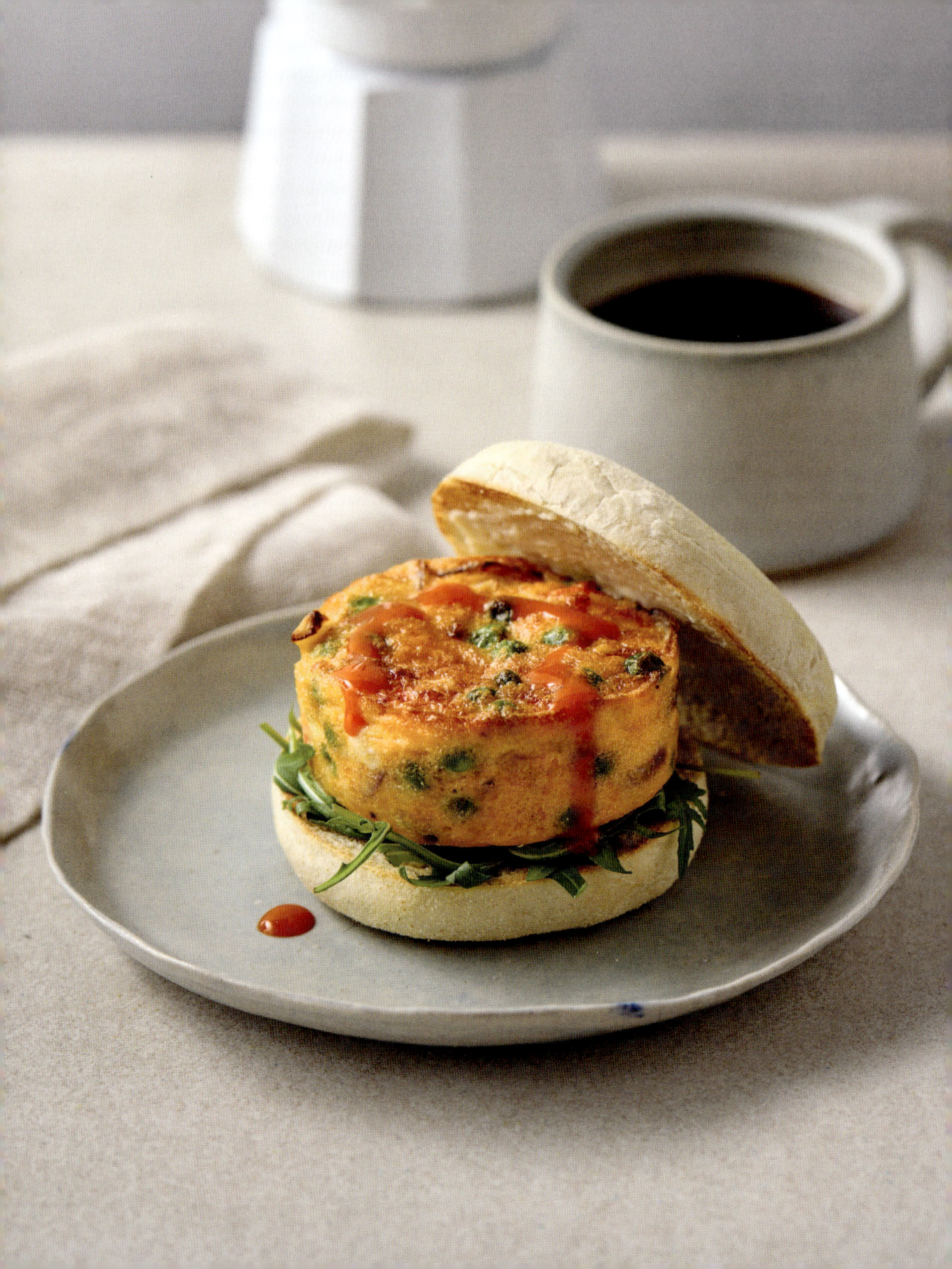

English Muffins with Frittata

Protein per serving: 22g **Kcals per serving: 356**

Serves 4

Prep + cook time: 25 minutes (35 minutes for a 20cm/8in frittata)

- ½ red onion, thinly sliced
- ½ red pepper, finely chopped
- 50g (generous ⅓ cup) frozen peas
- 70g (⅔ cup) grated Cheddar
- 15g (2 tbsp) pre-grated mozzarella
- 5 large eggs
- 4 English muffins
- handful of rocket (optional)
- salt and freshly ground black pepper
- vegetable or olive oil cooking spray

To serve (optional):

hot sauce

1 Preheat the oven to 190°C (170°C fan/375°F/Gas 5).

2 Grease four individual round tins or line a 20cm (8in) cake tin with baking parchment then set aside.

3 To a bowl, add the onion, red pepper, peas, Cheddar, and mozzarella. Crack the eggs into the bowl, season, then mix well.

4 Divide the egg mixture among the four individual tins, and cook for 20 minutes until set and a skewer comes out clean when inserted. Increase the cooking time to 30 minutes if using a single 20cm (8in) cake tin.

5 Meanwhile, cut the muffins in half and toast them. Arrange the rocket on the bottom halves, if using.

6 Tip the frittatas out onto a board (if using a 20cm/8in tin, cut the frittata into four pieces) and place on the bottom half of each muffin.

7 Splash over some hot sauce, if using, put the muffin lids on, and serve.

Keep it: Great hot or cold – once cooked these frittatas will keep in the fridge for 3 days.

Cheese is a bone-strengthening win alongside fibre-boosting veggies in this protein-packed dish.

Mixed Berry Baked Oats

Protein per serving: 17g **Kcals per serving: 401**

Serves 4

Prep + cook time: 45 minutes

- 2 bananas
- 220g (2⅓ cups) rolled oats
- 140ml (⅔ cup) milk
- 2 large eggs
- 130g (scant ⅔ cup) Greek yogurt
- 60ml (¼ cup) maple syrup
- 150g (5¼oz) frozen mixed berries
- butter, for greasing

1 Preheat the oven to 200°C (180°C fan/ 400°F/Gas 6). Grease and line a 18 x 23cm (7 x 9in) baking pan.

2 Add the bananas to a bowl and mash with a fork. Add the remaining ingredients and mix well until combined.

3 Transfer to the greased baking pan and smooth down with a spatula. Bake for 40 minutes until golden.

4 Leave to cool in the pan, then cut into bars.

Swap it: Bananas on their own would work well here; just leave out the berries and double the quantity of bananas.

Oats are a fantastic source of wholegrains. Alongside the richly coloured berries, this high-protein breakfast is protective for our heart health.

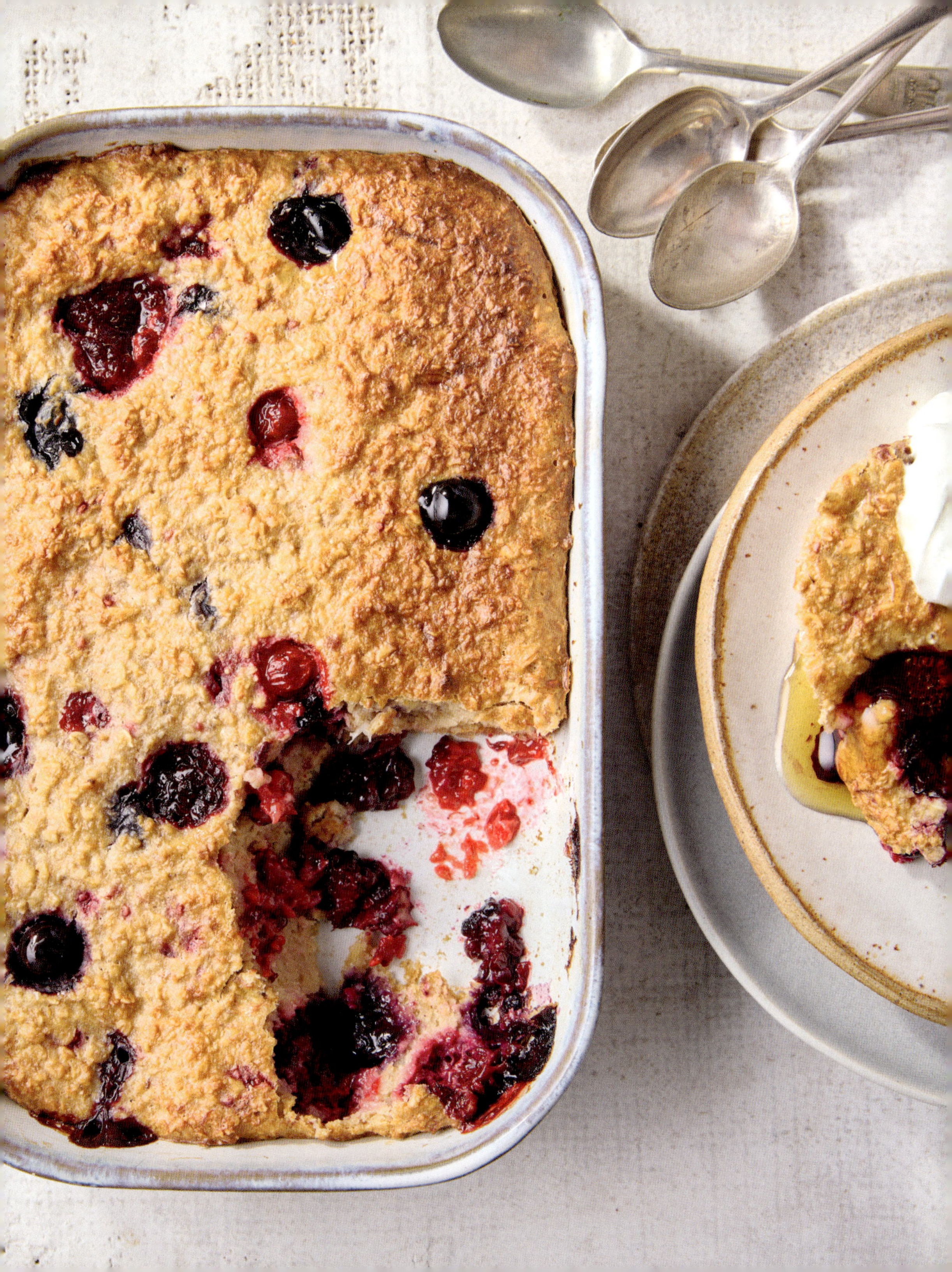

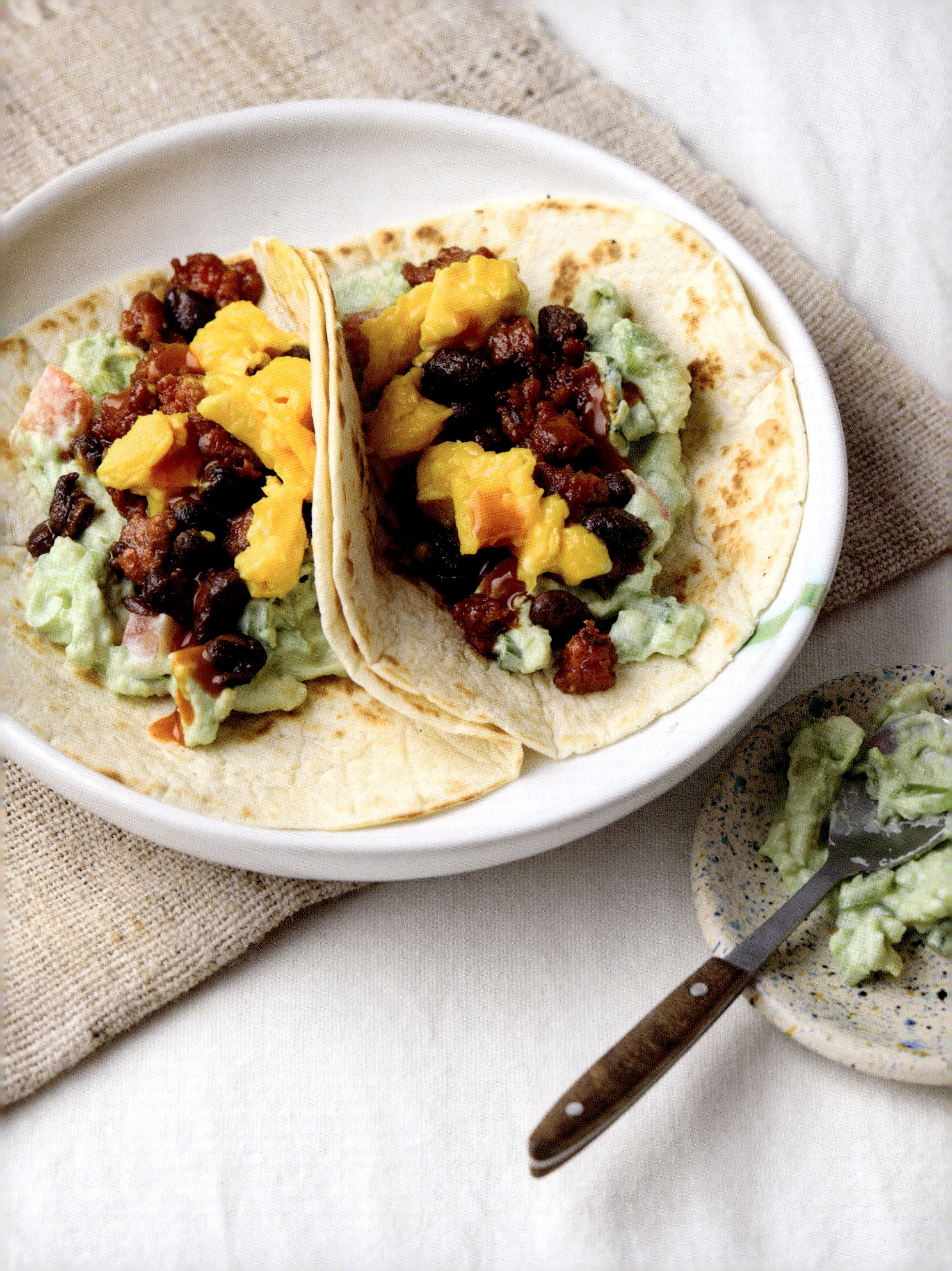

Breakfast Tacos

Protein per serving: 47g **Kcals per serving: 936**

Serves 4

Prep + cook time: 15 minutes

- 1 tbsp extra virgin olive oil
- 300g (10½oz) cooking chorizo, finely chopped
- 400g (14oz) can of black beans, drained and rinsed
- 2 avocados
- 2 tbsp Greek yogurt
- 2 spring onions, finely chopped
- 1 green chilli, deseeded and finely chopped
- 1 large tomato, roughly chopped
- 8 eggs
- 8 small tortilla wraps
- salt and freshly ground black pepper

To serve (optional):

- hot sauce
- lime juice

These tacos pack a nutritional punch with fibre and healthy fats from the black beans and avocados.

1 Add the olive oil to a pan, then set over a medium heat. Add the chorizo, then fry for about 5 minutes. Add the black beans, then fry for a further 2 minutes until the chorizo turns a dark brown and the beans have warmed through. Transfer to a bowl and set aside. Keep the pan for the eggs.

2 Meanwhile, in a bowl, lightly mash the avocado and Greek yogurt with a fork. Add the spring onions, green chilli, and tomato, then season with salt and freshly ground black pepper. Mix well and set aside.

3 Crack the eggs into a bowl, season with salt and freshly ground black pepper, and whisk.

4 Put the pan that the chorizo was cooked in back over a low heat. Add the eggs, and let them cook for 20 seconds before gently folding them. Cook for a further 2 minutes until softly set and runny in places.

5 Meanwhile, warm the tortillas in a frying pan or microwave.

6 To serve, spoon the avocado mix onto the tacos. Top with the chorizo and black beans, followed by the eggs, and serve with hot sauce and a squeeze of lime juice, if liked.

Swap it: Simply leave out the chorizo to make this veggie. To make this vegan, leave out the yogurt and swap the eggs out for some crumbled tofu.

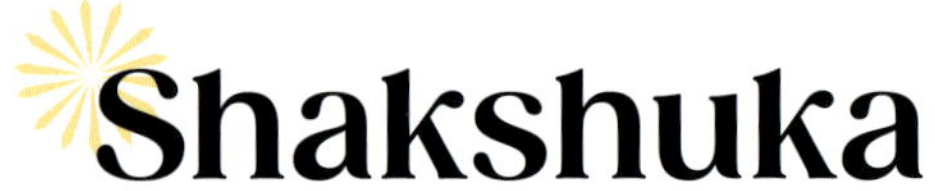

Shakshuka

Protein per serving: 26g **Kcals per serving: 550**

Serves 2

Prep + cook time: 15 minutes

- 1 tbsp extra virgin olive oil
- 1 red pepper, thinly sliced
- ½ onion, thinly sliced
- 300ml (1¼ cup) passata
- 2 tsp harissa
- 2 large eggs
- 100g (3½oz) feta
- handful of coriander, roughly chopped
- salt and freshly ground black pepper

To serve:

- lime wedges
- pitta breads

1 Set a pan for which you have a lid over a low-medium heat, then add the olive oil, pepper, and onion. Cook, uncovered, for 5 minutes until softened.

2 Add in the passata and harissa, then season with salt and freshly ground black pepper. Cook for 2 minutes until the sauce has reduced slightly.

3 Make two small wells in the sauce and crack an egg into each well. Cover the pan with the lid and cook for 5 minutes until the egg whites are set but the yolks are still runny.

4 Crumble over the feta and sprinkle over the coriander. Serve with lime wedges on the side and pitta breads for dipping.

Tip: This shakshuka makes for an impressive breakfast with just a handful of ingredients.

Passata is a rich source of lycopene, a powerful antioxidant linked to heart and skin health, which is more absorbable when cooked.

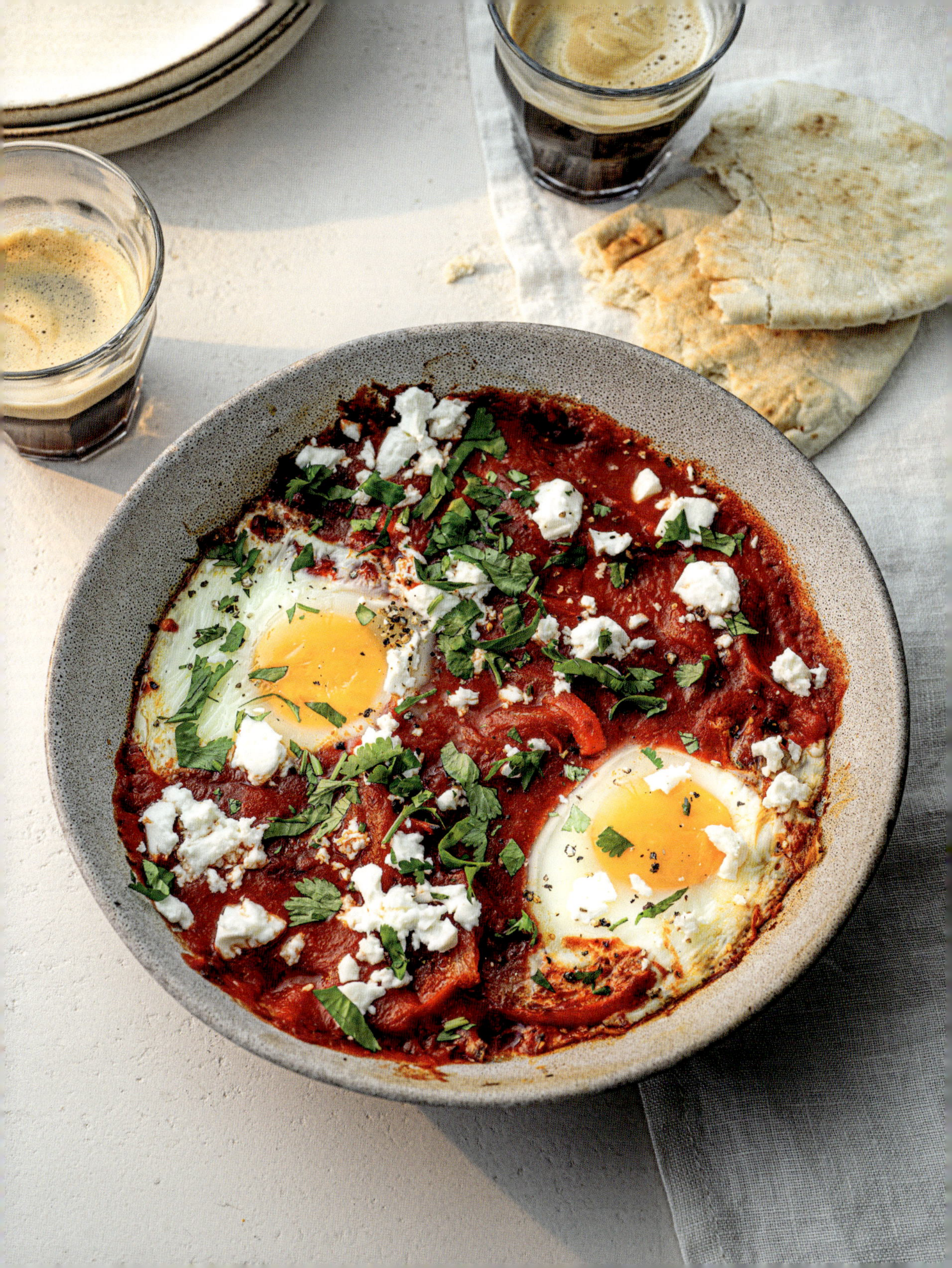

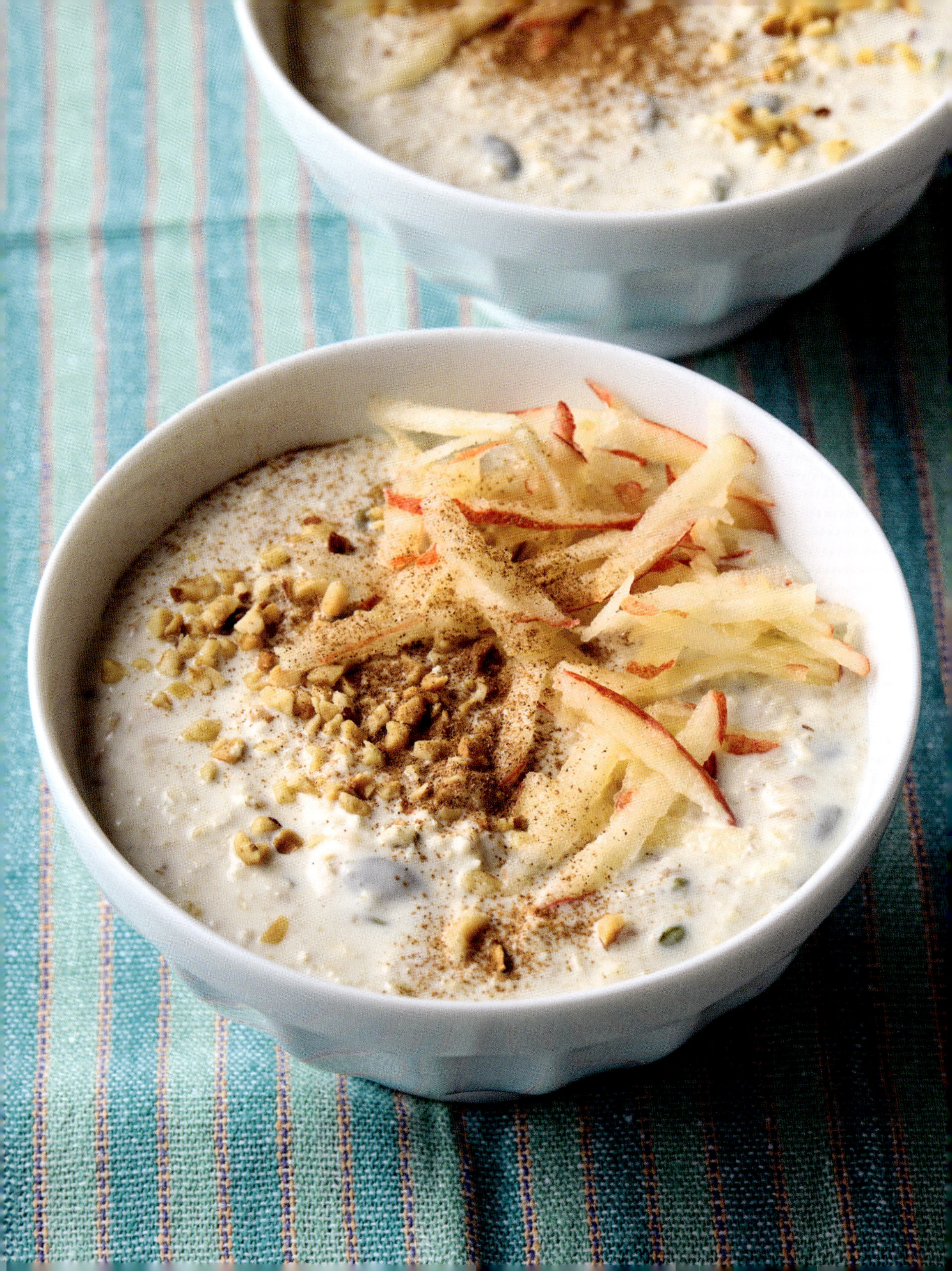

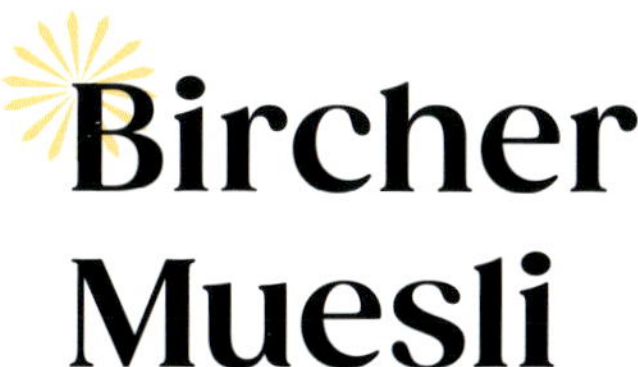

Bircher Muesli

Protein per serving: 16g **Kcals per serving: 476**

Serves 2

Prep time: 5 minutes, plus soaking overnight

- 60g (⅔ cup) jumbo porridge oats
- 2½ tbsp pumpkin seeds
- 2½ tbsp hazelnuts or brazil nuts, roughly chopped
- 100ml (6½ tbsp) apple juice
- 100g (scant ½ cup) Greek yogurt
- ¼ tsp ground cinnamon
- 1 apple, cored and grated
- salt

1 Add the oats, seeds, nuts, and apple juice to a bowl, then cover and leave to soak in the fridge overnight.

2 The next morning, add the Greek yogurt, cinnamon, and grated apple, along with a pinch of salt. Stir through and serve.

Swap it: To make this vegan, swap the yogurt for coconut yogurt.

The combination of protein-rich Greek yogurt with wholegrain oats will sustain you throughout the morning.

Scrambled Tofu

Protein per serving: 28g **Kcals per serving: 591**

Serves 2

Prep + cook time: 20 minutes

- 100g (3½oz) cherry tomatoes
- 2 tbsp extra virgin olive oil
- 280g (10oz) firm tofu
- ½ tsp ground turmeric
- ½ tsp smoked paprika
- 2 tbsp milk
- handful of oregano, leaves picked
- salt and freshly ground black pepper

To serve:

- 2 slices of sourdough
- 1 avocado, thinly sliced

1 Preheat the oven to 200°C (180°C fan/400°F/Gas 6).

2 Add the tomatoes to a baking dish, then drizzle over 1 tablespoon olive oil, and season with salt and freshly ground black pepper. Cook for 15 minutes until the tomatoes are bursting and look jammy, then set aside.

3 Meanwhile, set a pan over a low-medium heat, then add the remaining 1 tablespoon olive oil, the tofu, turmeric, paprika, and milk. Season with salt and lots of freshly ground black pepper, then cook for 5 minutes. Add the fresh oregano, then mix well and set aside.

4 Toast the sourdough.

5 Divide the tofu over both slices of toast, top with the tomatoes and serve with avocado on the side.

Swap it: To make this vegan, swap out the milk for a vegan alternative. Add a tablespoon of nutritional yeast, if liked, at the same time as the milk for extra flavour.

Tofu is a brilliant source of plant-based protein, providing all nine essential amino acids. Calcium-set varieties of firm tofu will also give your diet a bone-supporting boost.

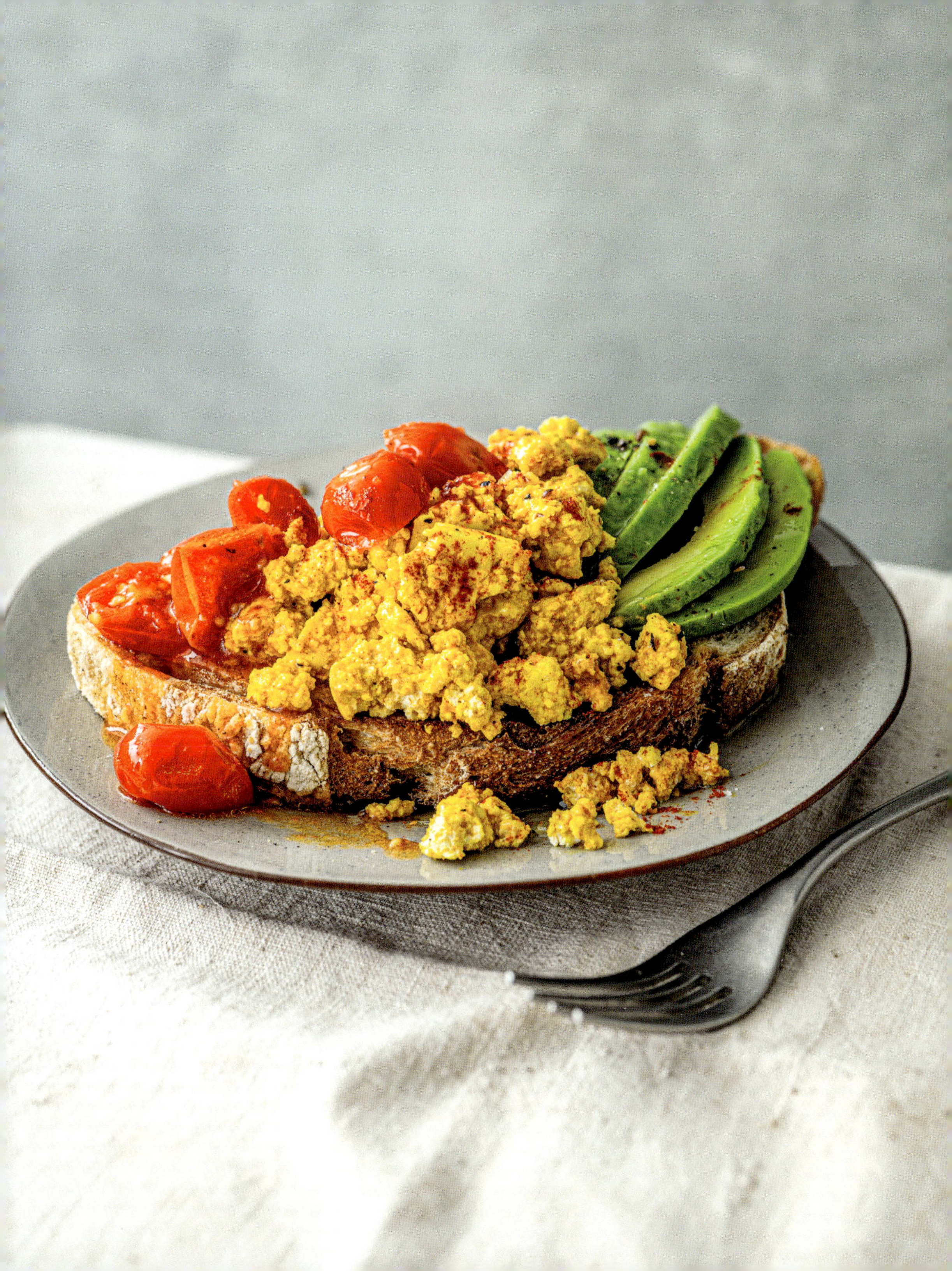

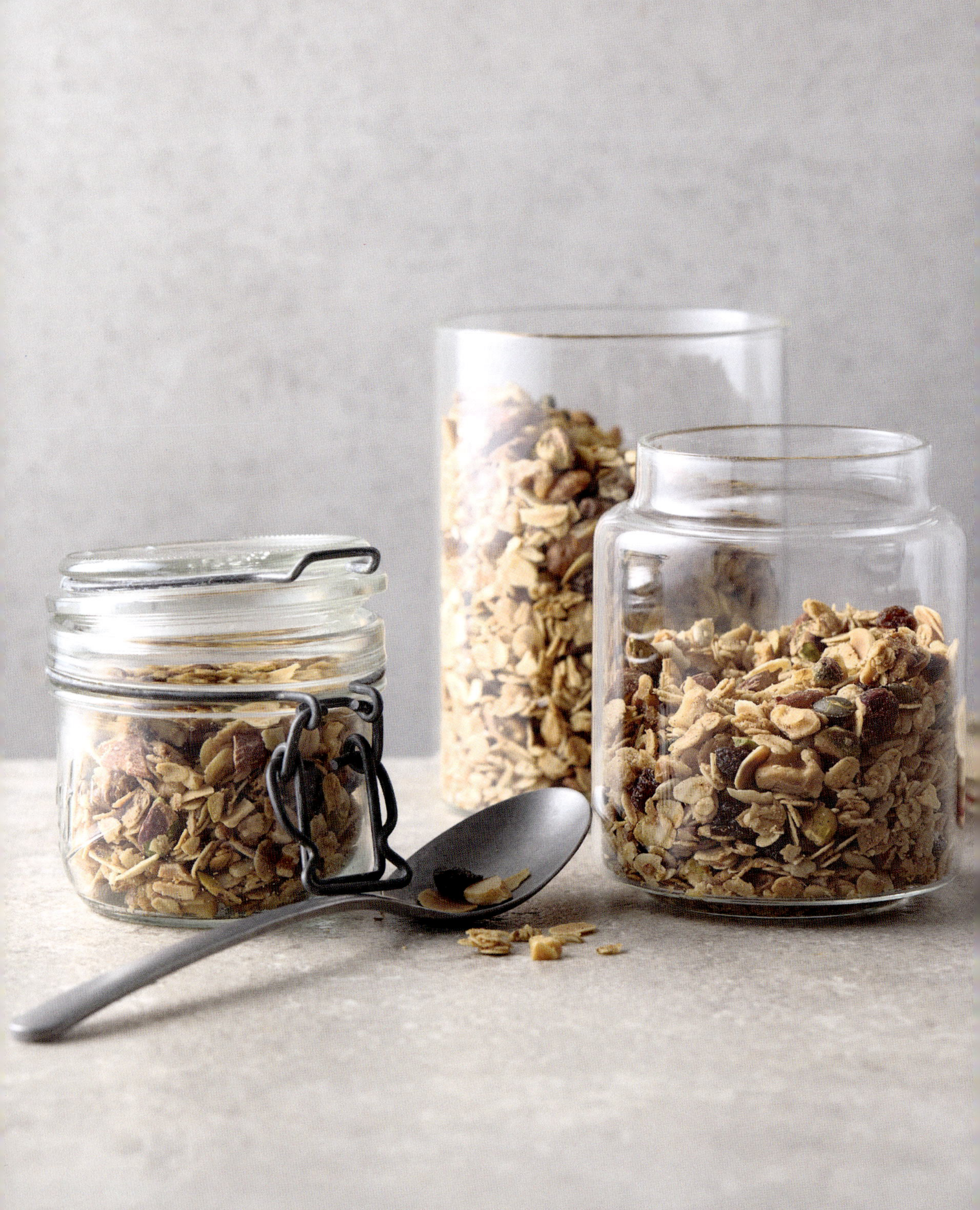

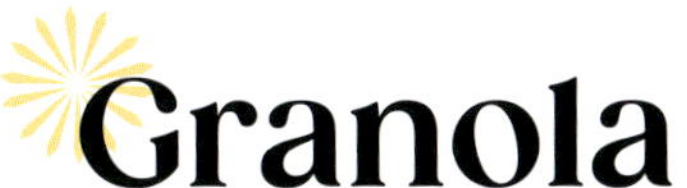

Granola

Protein per serving: 13g **Kcals per serving: 413**

Serves 6

Prep + cook time: 30 minutes

- 200g (generous 2 cups) jumbo oats
- 150g (generous 1 cup) mixed nuts, such almonds, walnuts, and pistachios
- 2½ tbsp pumpkin or sunflower seeds
- 1 tsp ground cinnamon
- 1 tsp ground ginger
- 50ml (3½ tbsp) maple syrup
- 2 tbsp coconut oil, melted
- 3 tbsp flaked almonds
- 2 tbsp raisins

1 Preheat the oven to 170°C (150°C fan/325°F/Gas 3).

2 Combine the oats, nuts, seeds, cinnamon, and ginger in a bowl. Add the maple syrup and coconut oil, then mix well.

3 Spread the granola out onto two baking sheets, then cook for 25 minutes, stirring at regular intervals.

4 Remove both trays from the oven, then add the flaked almonds and raisins. Leave to cool, then put in an airtight container.

Keep it: Store in an airtight container for up to 1 month.

Almonds help lower cholesterol, walnuts provide heart-healthy omega-3s, and pistachios support gut health with fibre and antioxidants.

Porridge with Nut Butter

Protein per serving: 14g **Kcals per serving: 393**

Serves 4

Prep + cook time: 10 minutes

- 200g (generous 2 cups) porridge oats
- 300ml (1¼ cups) milk
- 2 bananas, sliced
- 2 tbsp sesame seeds
- 60g (¼ cup) nut butter of choice (or see p28)
- salt

1 Into a large saucepan combine the porridge oats, milk, 500ml (2 cups) water, and 1 sliced banana. Cook over a medium heat until creamy, then stir through a pinch of salt.

2 Divide among four bowls, and top with the remaining banana slices, the sesame seeds, and the nut butter.

Tip: Mix in a tablespoon of tahini, if you have it, for an extra nutty hit.

Making porridge with milk instead of water is a simple way to boost its protein content and overall nutritional quality.

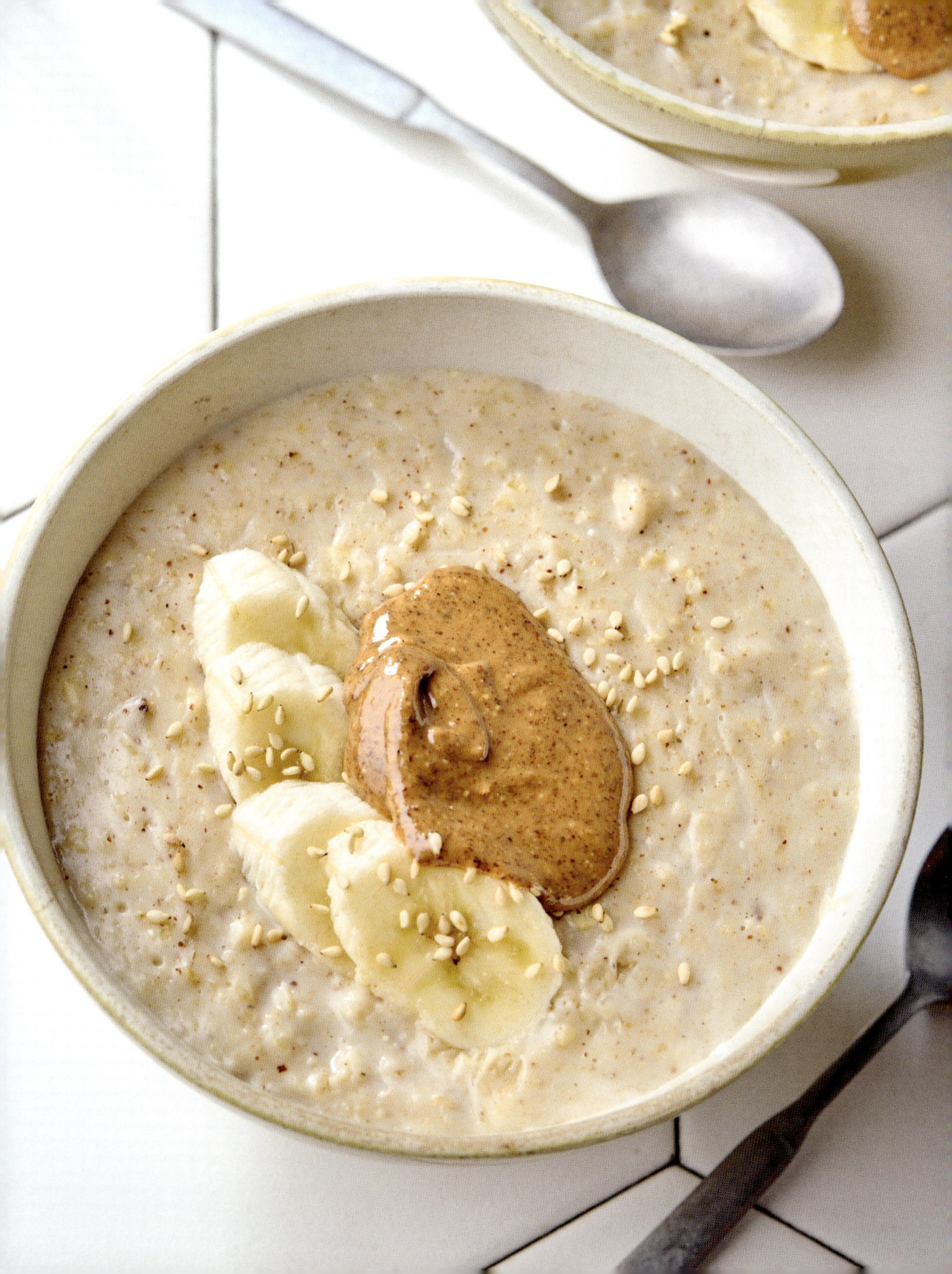

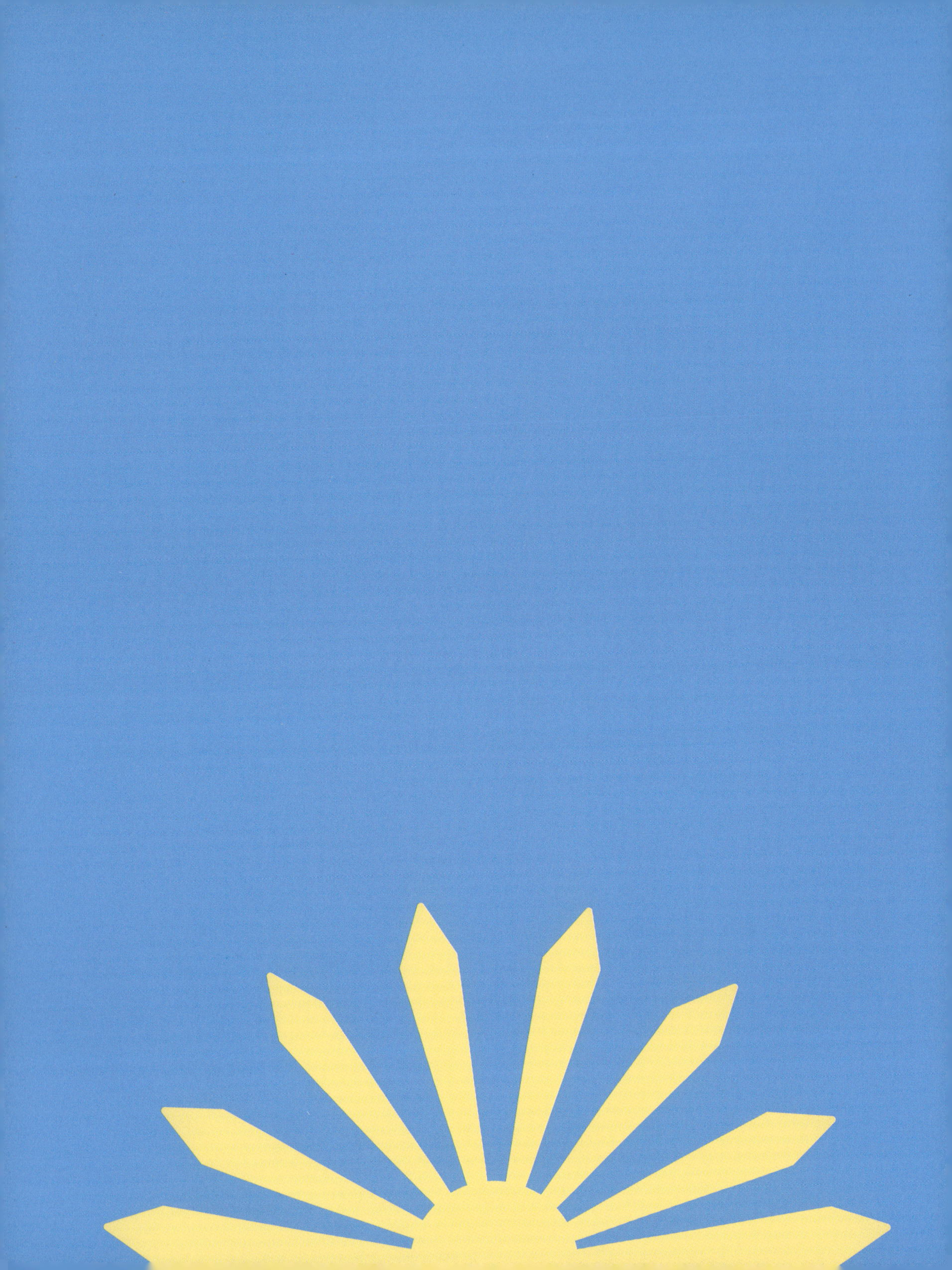

Protein-packed Lunches

These luscious lunches are loaded with protein to fuel the body. They will keep you full and energized throughout the afternoon. No more post-lunch slump at your desk! Many of the dishes can be prepped ahead of time for convenience – just make sure you store any dressings separately, and drizzle on when you're ready to enjoy.

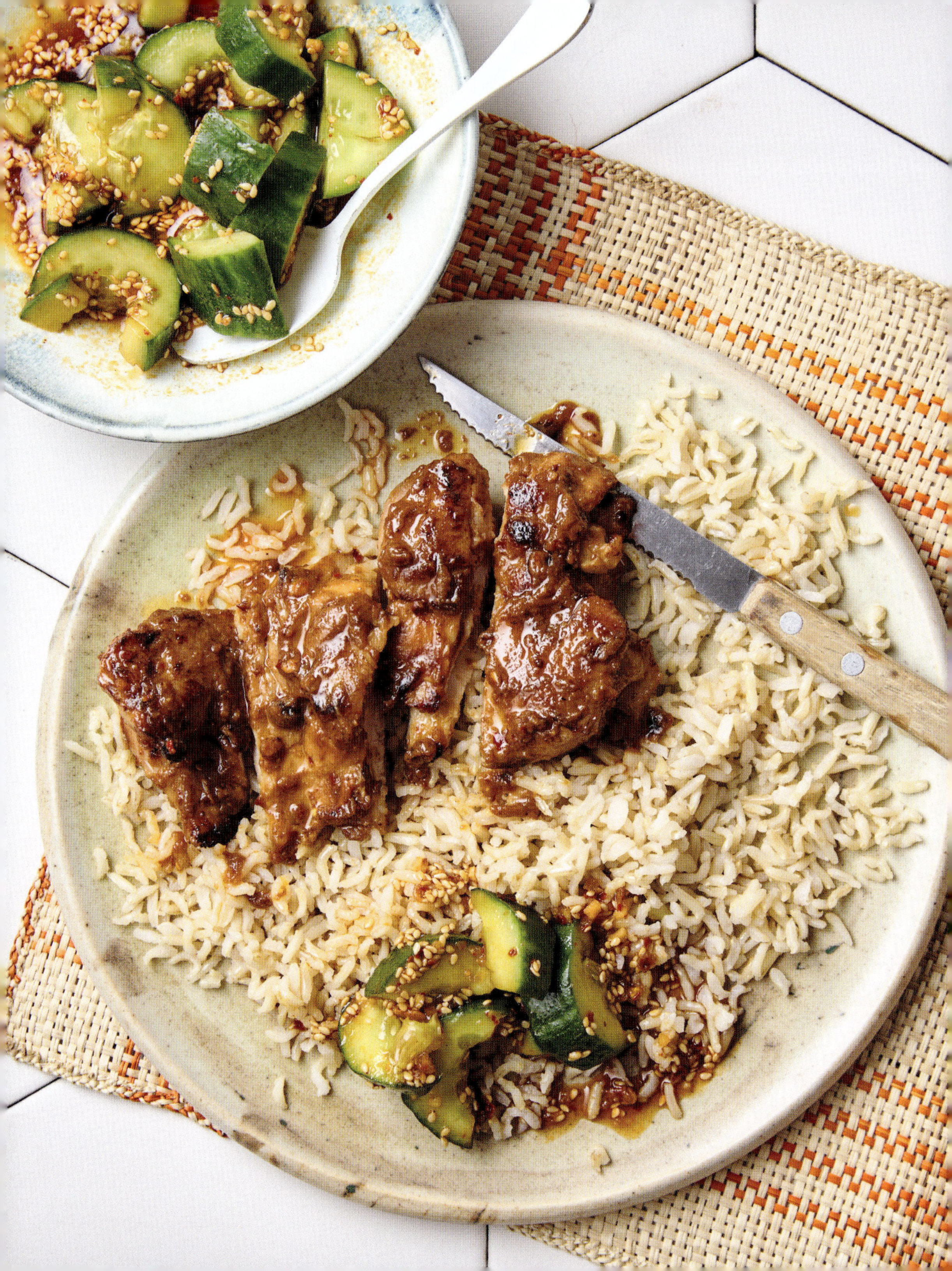

Miso Chicken with Smacked Cucumber

Protein per serving: 58g **Kcals per serving: 902**

Serves 2

Prep + cook time: 15 minutes, plus marinating

- 4 boneless, skinless chicken thighs
- 2 tbsp white miso paste
- 3 tbsp soy sauce
- 1 tbsp vegetable oil
- ½ cucumber
- 1 tbsp crispy chilli oil
- 1 clove of garlic, crushed
- 2cm (¾in) piece of ginger, peeled and finely chopped
- 1 tbsp fish sauce
- 1 tbsp sesame seeds
- 2 spring onions, finely chopped
- 250g (9oz) pouch of microwaveable brown rice

1 Put the chicken into a large bowl, then add the miso, 2 tablespoons soy sauce, and the vegetable oil. Mix together well until the chicken is coated, then set aside. If you have time, cover the bowl and leave to marinate in the fridge for up to 24 hours.

2 On a chopping board, bash the cucumber with a rolling pin until it splits, then roughly chop into 2cm (¾in) pieces. Put the cucumber into a bowl, then add the remaining 1 tablespoon soy sauce and the crispy chilli oil, along with the garlic, ginger, fish sauce, sesame seeds, and spring onions. Mix well and set aside.

3 Heat a griddle pan and set over a high heat. Once hot, add the chicken and cook for about 10 minutes, turning halfway through, until the chicken is nicely charred and cooked through.

4 Meanwhile, heat the rice pouch in the microwave according to the packet instructions.

5 Serve the chicken with the rice and cucumber.

Swap it: This also works well with salmon or cod.

Chicken is a high-quality source of lean protein, especially when we choose cuts without the skin.

Ginger Chicken Congee

Protein per serving: 49g **Kcals per serving: 657**

Serves 2

Prep + cook time: 20 minutes

- 300g (10½oz) chicken mince
- 2 cloves of garlic, crushed
- 2cm (¾in) piece of ginger, finely chopped
- 1 tbsp oyster sauce
- 2 tbsp soy sauce
- 4 spring onions, finely chopped
- handful of coriander, roughly chopped
- 1 tbsp extra virgin olive oil
- 250g (9oz) pouch of microwaveable sticky rice
- 250ml (1 cup) vegetable stock
- 1 tbsp sesame oil
- 1 tbsp sesame seeds

1 To a bowl, add the chicken mince, garlic, ginger, oyster sauce, soy, half the spring onions, and half the coriander. Mix well, then mould into 20g (⅔oz) meatballs. Set aside.

2 Set a saucepan over a medium-high heat and add the olive oil. Once hot, add the meatballs, in a single layer, and cook for 10 minutes until golden on all sides and cooked through. Remove and set aside.

3 Squeeze the packet of rice to loosen, then add the rice to the saucepan. Add the vegetable stock, and cook for around 5 minutes until the rice has softened.

4 Divide the congee between two bowls, top with the chicken, remaining spring onion, and remaining coriander. Drizzle over the sesame oil and sprinkle over the sesame seeds.

Swap it: To make this veggie replace the chicken balls with roasted butternut squash or mushrooms.

Chicken mince is a high-protein, lower-fat alternative to beef mince, and is incredibly versatile. Here it is paired with the digestive benefits of ginger.

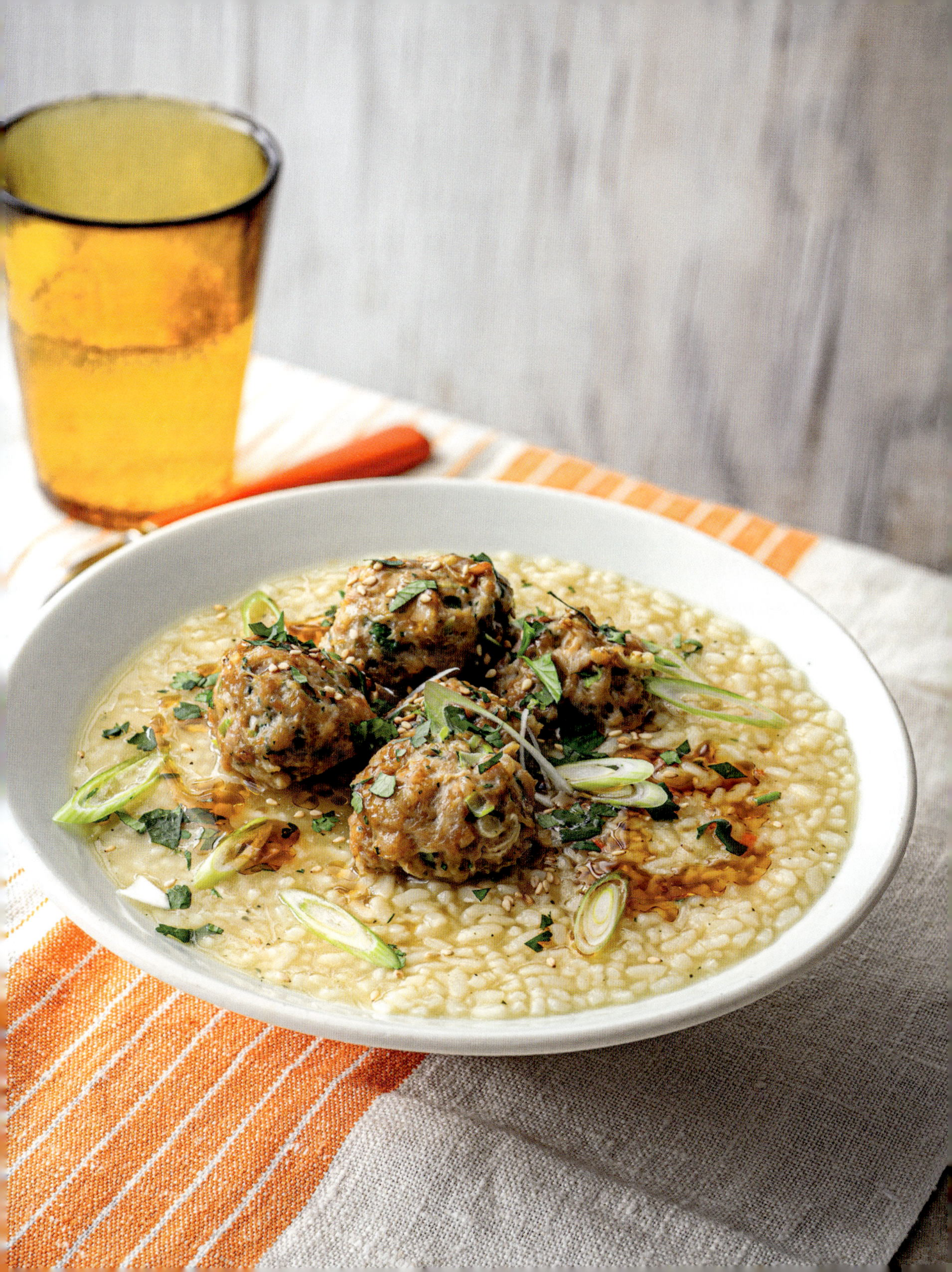

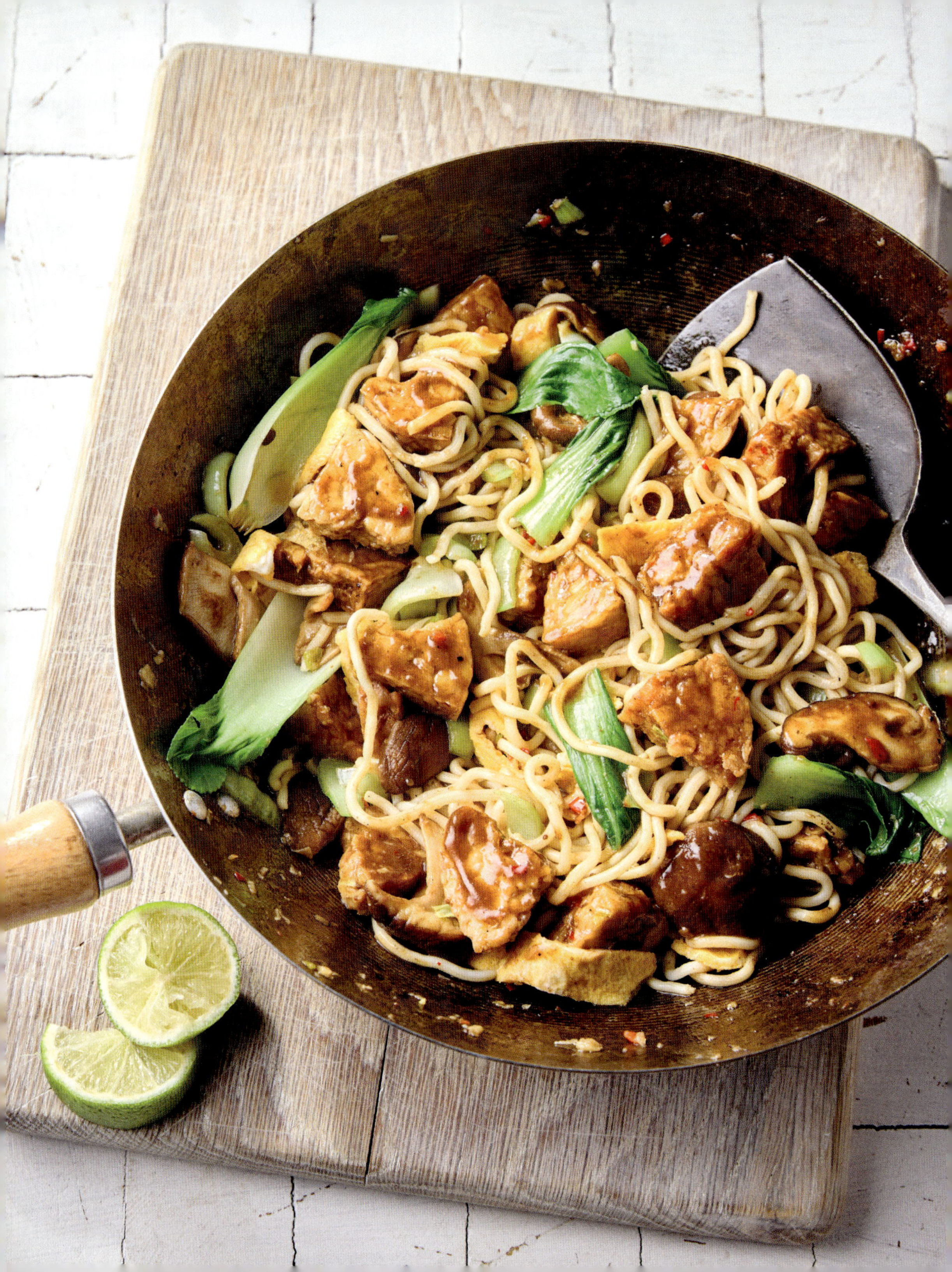

Tempeh and Mushroom Stir Fry

Protein per serving: 53g **Kcals per serving: 886**

Serves 2

Prep + cook time: 10 minutes

- 2 large eggs
- 2 tbsp vegetable oil
- 200g (7oz) tempeh, cut into 2cm (¾in) cubes
- 120g (4oz) shiitake or chestnut mushrooms
- 2 cloves of garlic, crushed
- 2cm (¾in) piece of ginger, finely chopped
- ½ red chilli, deseeded and finely chopped
- 195g (7oz) black bean sauce
- 200g (7oz) pak choi, leaves separated and stalks roughly chopped
- 200g (7oz) straight-to-wok medium egg noodles
- juice of 1 lime

1 Crack the eggs into a small bowl, whisk well, and set aside.

2 Add the oil to a wok or frying pan over a high heat. Add the tempeh and mushrooms and fry for 2 minutes until both are golden. Add the garlic, ginger, and chilli, and cook for 30 seconds.

3 Add the black bean sauce, pak choi stalks, and noodles, along with a splash of water. Cook for 1 minute until the noodles have softened.

4 Push all the ingredients to one side of the pan, and pour the eggs into the empty space. Let the eggs sit for 30 seconds until slightly set, then mix through the noodles. Add the pak choi leaves and the lime juice, then cook until the leaves are just wilted, then serve.

Tip: Prawns would also work well here.

Tempeh offers protein and fibre, while mushrooms provide antioxidants, B vitamins, and vitamin D.

Tuscan-style Soup

Protein per serving: 20g **Kcals per serving: 360**

Serves 4

Prep + cook time: 20 minutes

- 1 tbsp extra virgin olive oil
- 1 carrot, peeled and finely chopped
- 1 onion, finely chopped
- 1 celery stick, finely chopped
- 2 cloves of garlic, crushed
- 2 x 400g (14oz) cans of cannellini beans, drained and rinsed
- 1 tbsp tomato purée
- 400g (14oz) can of cherry tomatoes
- 500ml (2 cups) vegetable stock
- 100g (3½oz) kale, stalks removed and roughly chopped
- handful of basil leaves
- 3 slices of slightly stale seeded bread, cut into large chunks
- 1 tbsp red wine vinegar
- salt and freshly ground black pepper

1 Add the olive oil to a large saucepan and set over a medium-low heat. Add in the carrot, onion, celery, and garlic. Cook for 10 minutes until softened.

2 Add in the beans, tomato purée, cherry tomatoes, and vegetable stock. Cook over a medium heat until the sauce is reduced and thickened, but still soupy.

3 Add in the kale, basil, bread, and red wine vinegar. Season with salt and freshly ground black pepper, stir well so the kale wilts into the soup, and serve.

Swap it: Swap the cannellini beans for chickpeas or butter beans, if you prefer.

Soup can often be on the low side for protein, but in this recipe, protein is high thanks to the addition of cannellini beans.

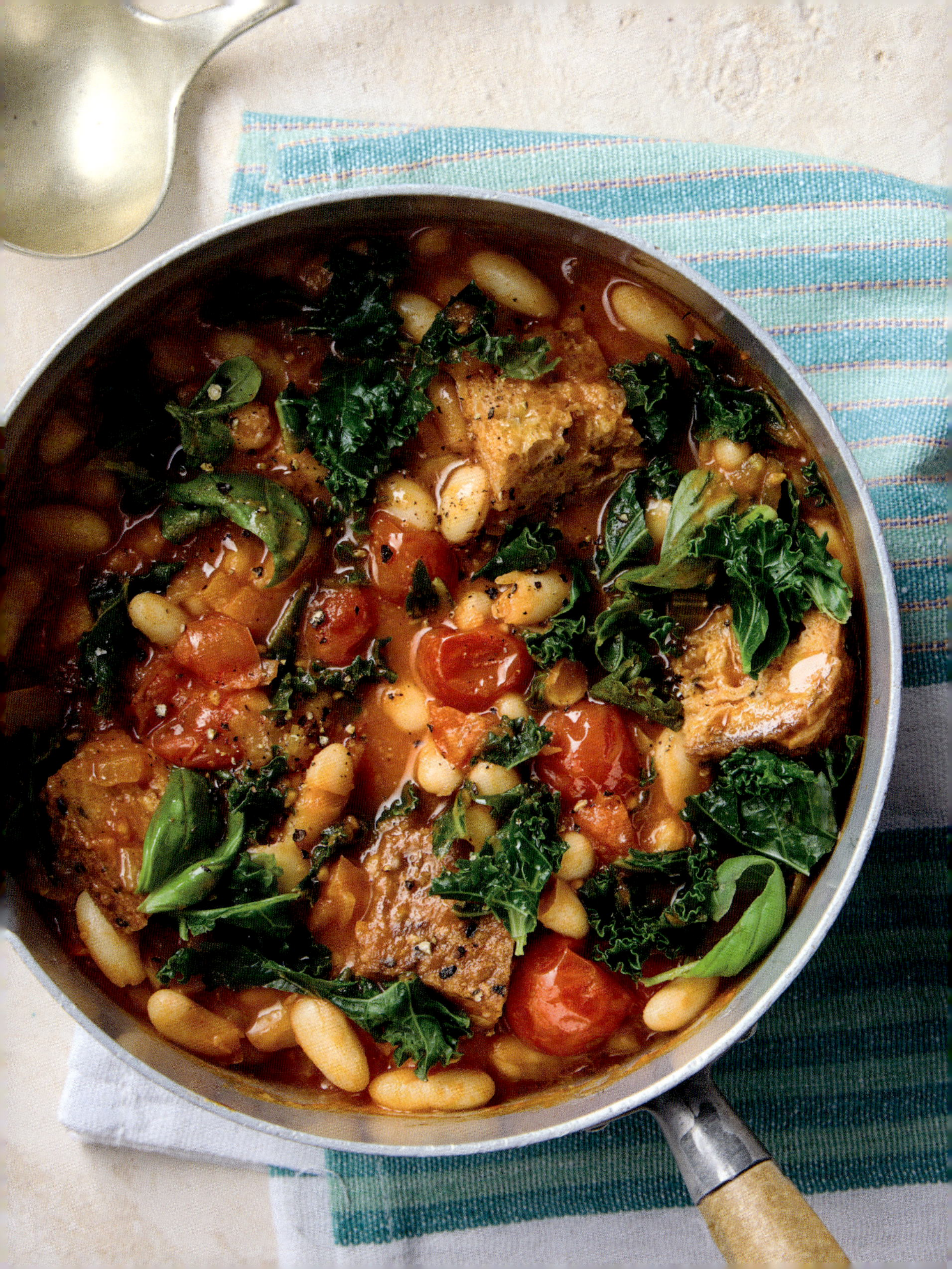

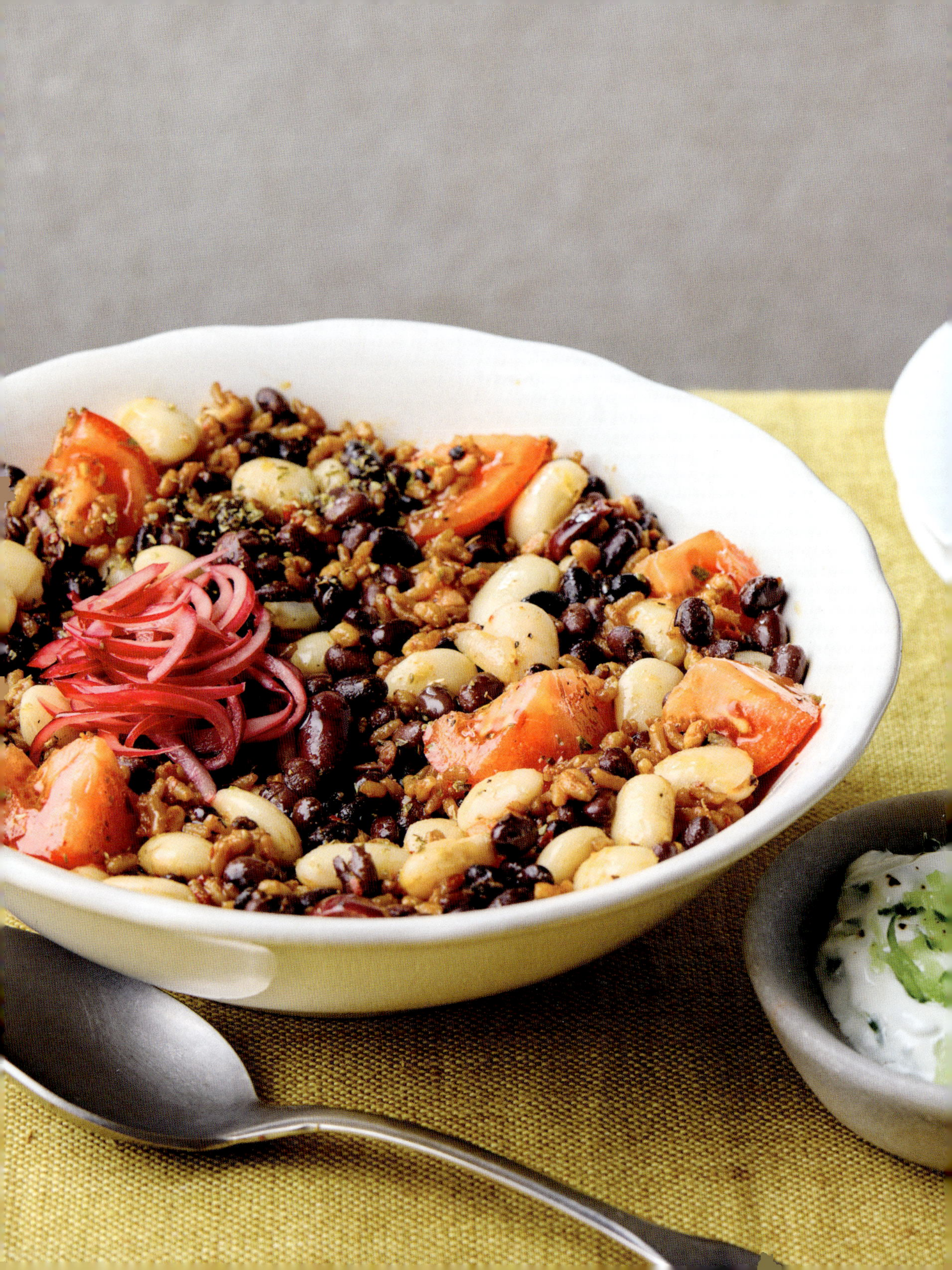

Greek Bean Salad

Protein per serving: 19g **Kcals per serving: 449**

Serves 4

Prep + cook time: 20 minutes

- ½ red onion, thinly sliced
- 2 tbsp red wine vinegar
- 400g (14oz) can of black beans, drained and rinsed
- 400g (14oz) can of butter beans, drained and rinsed
- 2 large tomatoes, roughly chopped
- 50g (½ cup) pitted black olives, roughly chopped
- 1 tbsp dried oregano
- 50ml (3½ tbsp) extra virgin olive oil
- 250g (9oz) pouch of microwaveable grains
- 150g (¾ cup) Greek yogurt
- ¼ cucumber, grated
- salt and freshly ground black pepper

To serve:

- 4 wholemeal pitta breads (optional)

1 To a small bowl, add the red onion, red wine vinegar, and a pinch of salt. Scrunch together with your hands, then set aside for 5 minutes to pickle lightly.

2 In a bowl, combine the black beans, butter beans, tomatoes, olives, oregano, and olive oil. Season with salt and freshly ground black pepper. Add in the pickled red onion, then mix well and set aside for 10 minutes to marinate.

3 Microwave the grain pouch according to the packet instructions and set aside.

4 To a small bowl, add the yogurt and cucumber. Season with salt and black pepper, then mix well and set aside.

5 To assemble, add the grain pouch to the bean bowl and stir. Serve with the cucumber yogurt and pittas on the side, if liked.

Swap it: To make this recipe vegan, swap the Greek yogurt for a vegan alternative.

Pulses are packed with plant protein, fibre, and slow-release carbs to support blood sugar balance and gut health.

Chicken Pesto Pasta

Protein per serving: 45g **Kcals per serving: 788**

Serves 4

Prep + cook time: 20 minutes

- 200g (7oz) wholewheat fusilli or penne
- 3 tbsp extra virgin olive oil
- 3 chicken breasts
- 200g (scant 1 cup) Greek yogurt
- 130g (⅔ cup) pesto
- grated zest and juice of 2 lemons
- 100g (1 cup) pitted green olives, roughly chopped
- 200g (7oz) jarred red peppers, sliced
- 2 x 400g (14oz) cans of chickpeas, drained and rinsed
- 60g (2oz) rocket
- salt and freshly ground black pepper

1 Fill a large saucepan with water, salt well, and bring to the boil. Once boiling, add the pasta and cook according to the packet instructions.

2 Meanwhile, set a griddle pan over a high heat. Drizzle 1 tablespoon olive oil over the chicken. Once the pan is hot, add the chicken and cook for about 10 minutes, turning halfway through, until cooked through. Remove from the pan, shred the chicken, and place into a large bowl.

3 Into a small bowl, combine the Greek yogurt, pesto, lemon zest, and lemon juice, then season with salt and freshly ground black pepper. Mix well and set aside.

4 Once the pasta is ready, drain, then add to the bowl with the chicken. Add the olives, peppers, chickpeas, rocket, and pesto yogurt, then season with salt and freshly ground black pepper. Mix well, then serve.

Swap it: This works well with a lentil-based pasta.

Chicken and chickpeas provide a powerful mix of lean animal and plant proteins, plus fibre and iron to support energy, fullness, and muscle health.

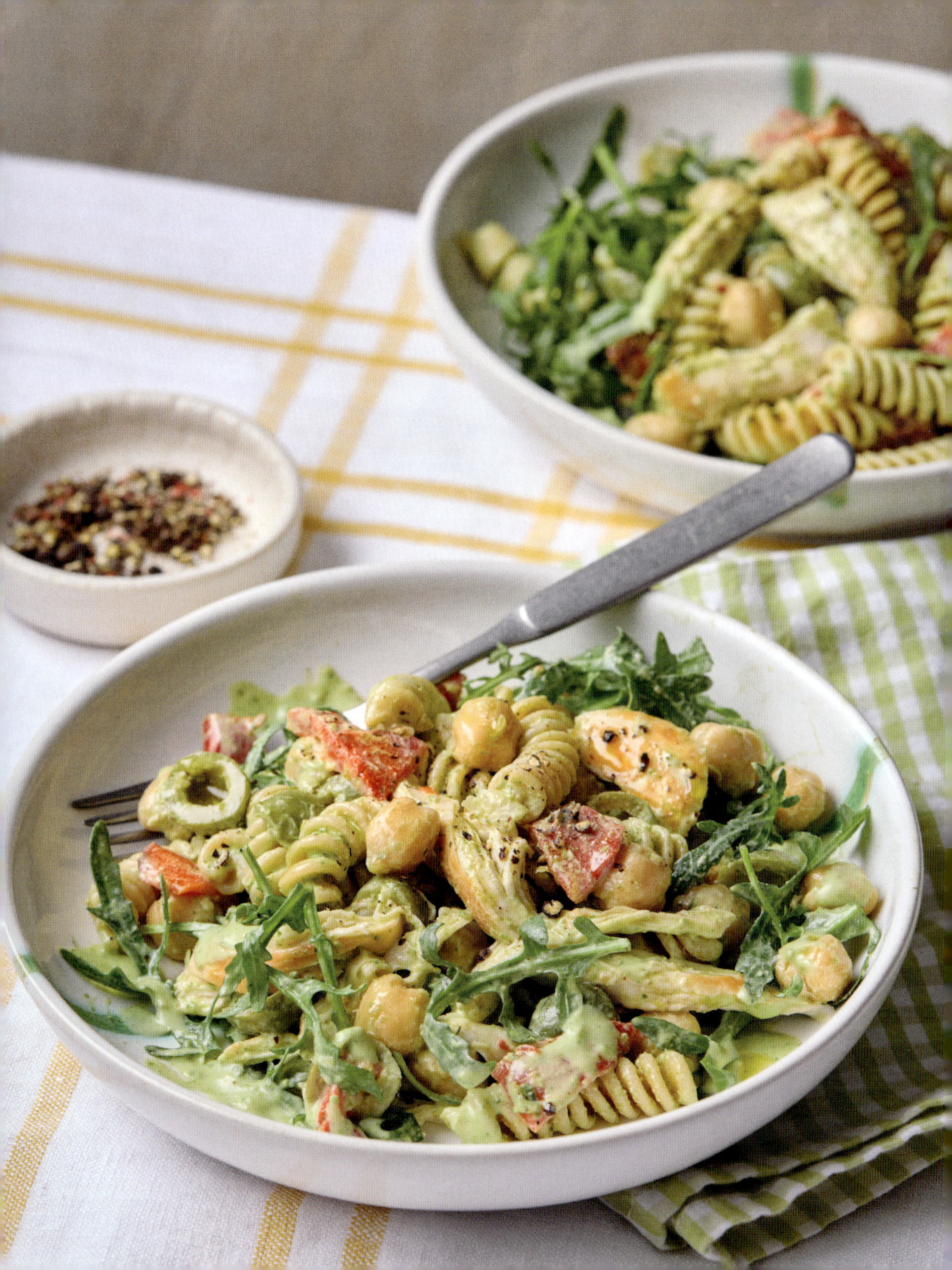

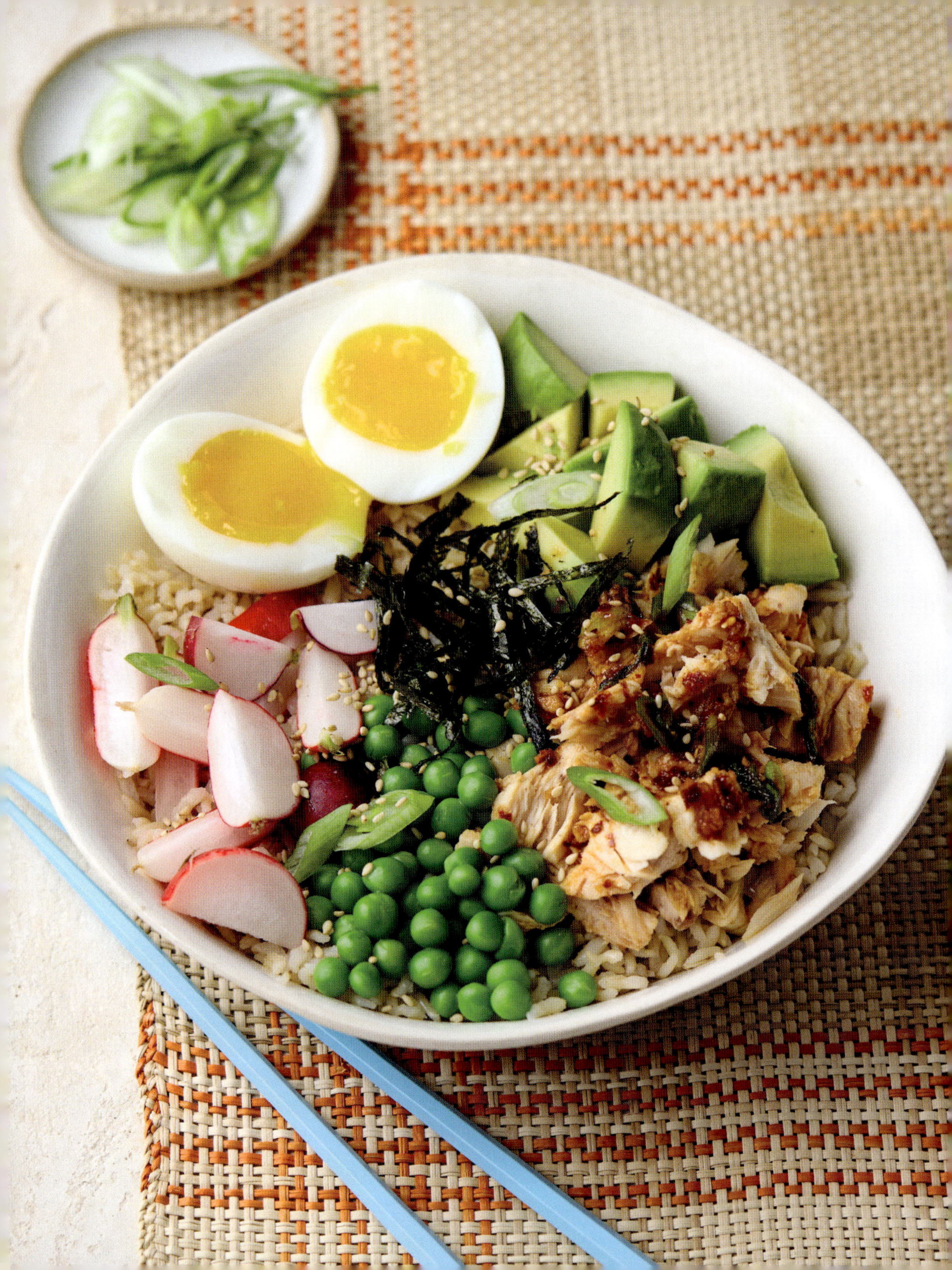

Spicy Tuna Sushi Bowl

Protein per serving: 35g **Kcals per serving: 584**

Serves 2

Prep + cook time: 15 minutes

- 2 large eggs
- 50g (1¾oz) radish, thinly sliced
- 1 tbsp rice wine vinegar
- 250g (9oz) pouch of microwaveable brown rice
- 145g (5oz) can of tuna, drained
- 1 tbsp crispy chilli oil
- 1 tbsp soy sauce
- 1 spring onion, finely chopped
- 1 avocado, cut into chunks
- 100g (¾ cup) frozen peas, defrosted
- 4 nori sheets, cut into thin strips
- 1 tbsp toasted sesame seeds
- salt

1 Fill a saucepan with water and bring to the boil. Once boiling, add the eggs to the pan and cook for 6 minutes. Remove the eggs, run them under cold water, and set aside.

2 Meanwhile, to a small bowl add the radish and rice wine vinegar, along with a pinch of salt, then set aside.

3 Microwave the rice pouch according to the packet instructions and set aside.

4 To a small bowl, add the tuna, crispy chilli oil, soy, and spring onion. Mix together, then set aside.

5 To assemble, divide the rice pouch between two bowls. Top with the tuna, avocado, and peas. Peel the eggs, cut them in half, and arrange them on top. Finish with the pickled radish, nori, and sesame seeds.

Swap it: This works really well with salmon or tofu, if you prefer them.

Tuna is a convenient source of protein. Choose tuna in spring water to keep the fat content down.

Green Lentil Prawn Salad

Protein per serving: 30g **Kcals per serving: 609**

Serves 2

Prep + cook time: 15 minutes

- ¼ red onion, thinly sliced
- 2 tbsp apple cider vinegar
- 3 tbsp extra virgin olive oil
- 1 small onion, finely chopped
- 2 cloves of garlic, crushed
- 165g (6oz) peeled raw king prawns
- 250g (9oz) pouch of microwaveable puy lentils
- 1 tsp Dijon mustard
- 1 tsp maple syrup
- 50g (1¾oz) radish, thinly sliced
- ¼ cucumber, roughly chopped
- 100g (3½oz) cherry tomatoes, halved
- 1 avocado, roughly chopped
- 70g (2½oz) baby spinach
- salt and freshly ground black pepper

1 To a small bowl, add the red onion, 1 tablespoon apple cider vinegar, and a pinch of salt. Scrunch together with your hands and set aside to pickle.

2 Heat 1 tablespoon olive oil in a frying pan over a low heat. Add the onion and garlic, and cook for a few minutes until the onion has softened. Add the prawns and cook until just pink. Set aside.

3 Microwave the lentil pouch according to the packet instructions, then set aside.

4 Meanwhile, to a small bowl add the remaining 2 tablespoons olive oil and 1 tablespoon apple cider vinegar, along with the Dijon mustard and maple syrup to make the dressing. Season with salt and pepper, whisk well, and set aside.

5 To a large bowl, add the lentils, prawns, radish, cucumber, tomatoes, avocado, and spinach. Stir in the dressing, and serve with the pickled red onion.

Swap it: Swap the lentils for any pouch of grains.

Together, prawns and green lentils combine lean protein, iron, and zinc with fibre and slow-release carbs.

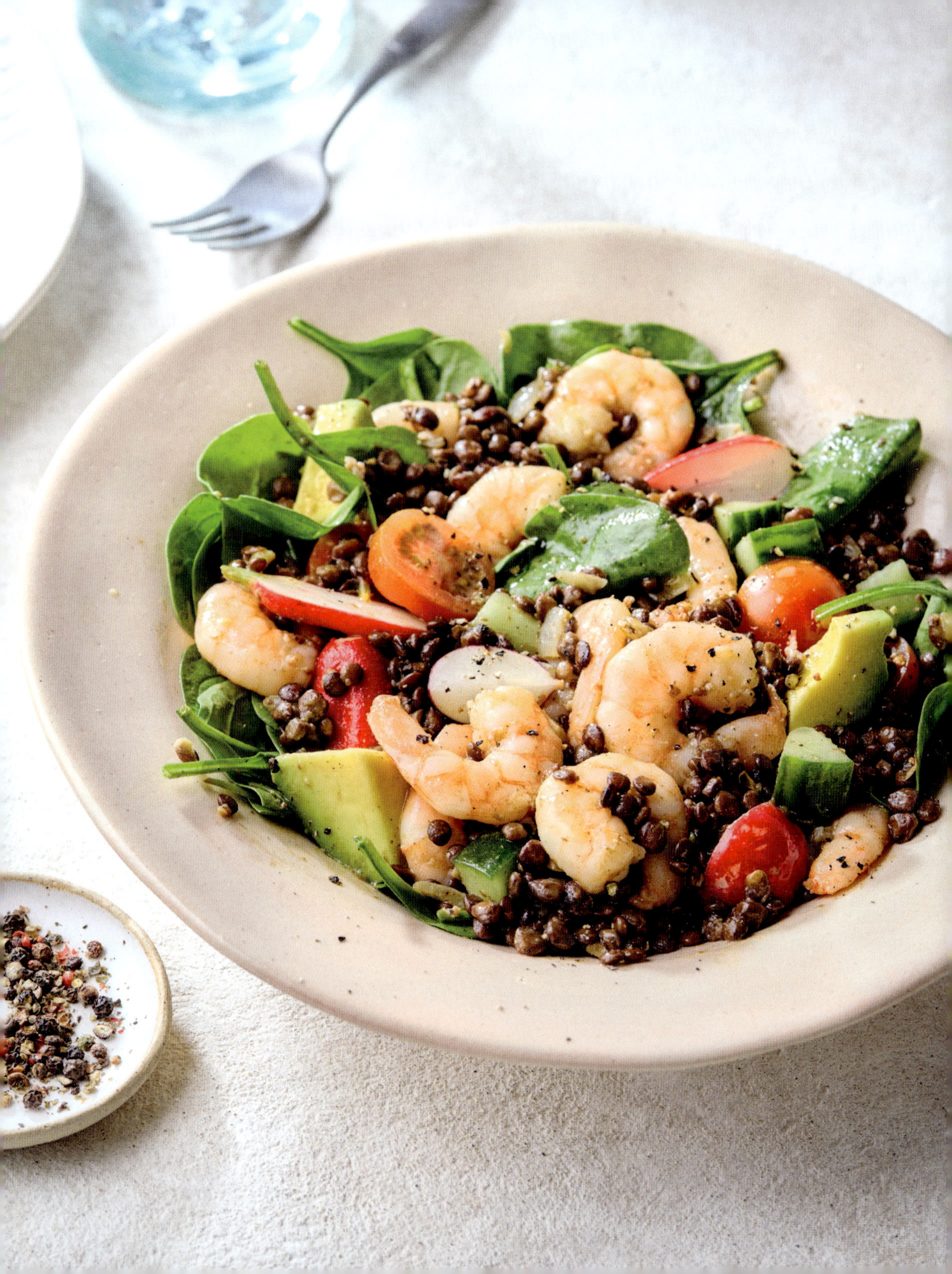

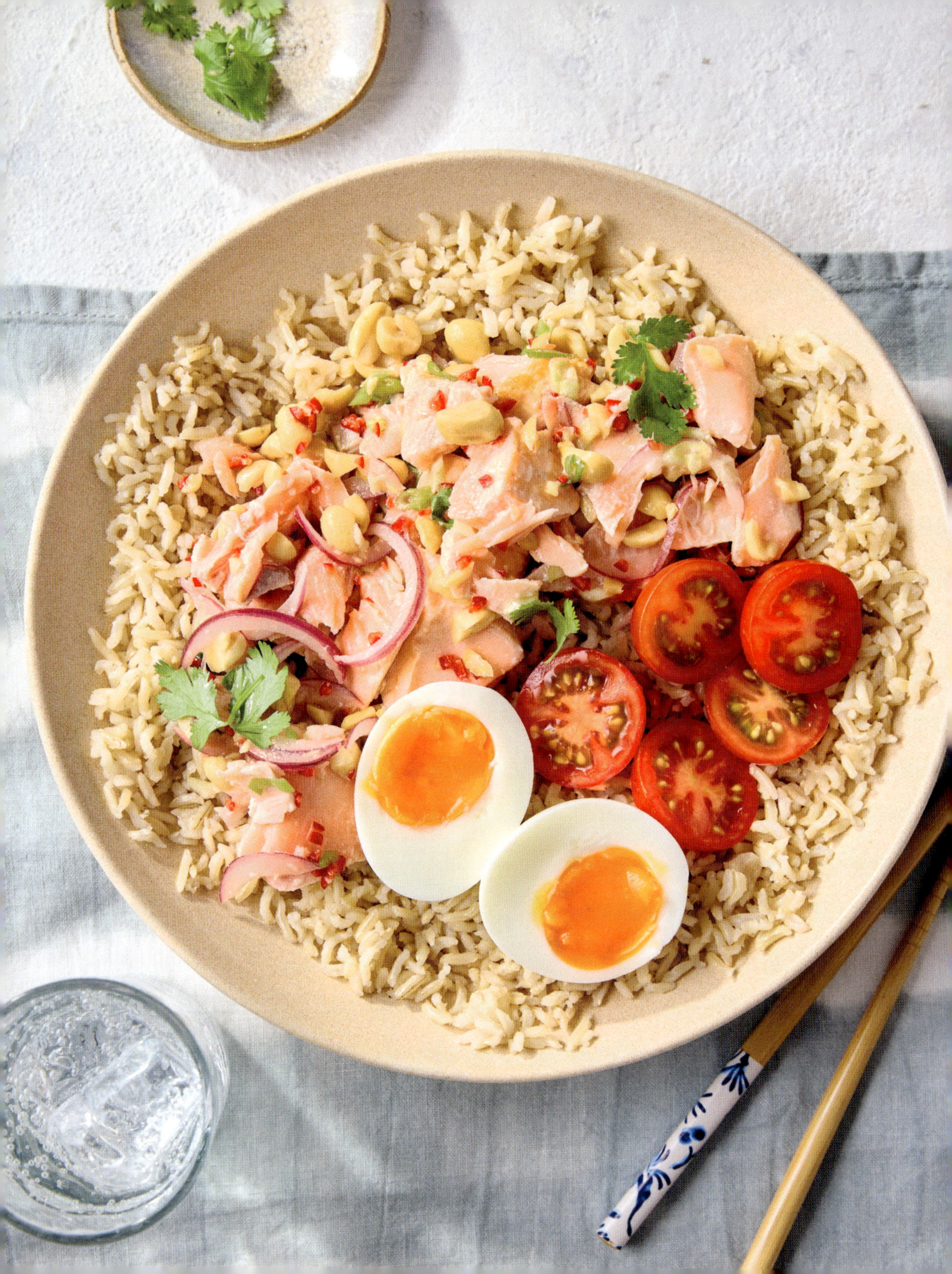

Salmon Rice Bowl

Protein per serving: 45g **Kcals per serving: 741**

Serves 2

Prep + cook time: 15 minutes

- 2 large eggs
- 2 tbsp fish sauce
- juice of 3 limes
- 1 tsp caster sugar
- 1 red chilli, deseeded and finely chopped
- ½ red onion, thinly sliced
- 40g (scant ⅓ cup) peanuts, roughly chopped
- handful of coriander, roughly chopped
- 2 spring onions, finely chopped
- 1 tbsp vegetable oil
- 2 salmon fillets
- 250g (9oz) pouch of microwaveable brown basmati rice
- 50g (1¾oz) cherry tomatoes, halved

1 Fill a saucepan with water and bring to the boil. Once boiling, add the eggs to the pan and cook for 7 minutes. Drain, run under cold water to stop the cooking process, and set aside.

2 Meanwhile, to a bowl add the fish sauce, lime juice, sugar, chilli, red onion, peanuts, coriander, and spring onions. Mix well, then set aside.

3 Add the vegetable oil to a frying pan, then set over a medium heat. Once hot, add the salmon to the pan, skin-side down, and fry for 2 minutes on each side until cooked through. Remove the salmon from the pan, then flake the fish into large pieces. Add to the fish sauce dressing, mix well, and set aside.

4 Heat the rice pouch in the microwave according to the packet instructions.

5 Divide the rice between two bowls and top with the salmon. Peel and halve the eggs, then add to the bowls along with the tomatoes.

Swap it: This would also work well with tuna.

Salmon provides EPA and DHA, the anti-inflammatory fats that support heart health, brain function, and mood regulation.

Chipotle Steak Bowl

Protein per serving: 33g **Kcals per serving: 587**

Serves 4

Prep + cook time: 30 minutes

- 300g (10½oz) sweet potatoes, peeled and cut into 3cm (1¼in) pieces
- 3 tbsp extra virgin olive oil
- 200g (7oz) frozen sweetcorn, defrosted
- handful of coriander, roughly chopped
- 1 large tomato, roughly chopped
- 400g (14oz) can of kidney beans, drained and rinsed
- juice of 3 limes
- 2 tbsp chipotle paste
- 1 tbsp honey
- 3 sirloin steaks, cut into 4cm (1½in) chunks
- 2 avocados, cut into chunks
- ½ iceberg lettuce, finely shredded
- salt and freshly ground black pepper

Lean steak cuts are readily available and a fantastic source of protein for the body.

1 Preheat the oven to 200°C (180°C fan/400°F/Gas 6).

2 Put the sweet potatoes onto a large baking tray and drizzle over 1 tablespoon olive oil. Season with salt and freshly ground black pepper, then cook in the oven for 15–20 minutes until softened. Set aside.

3 Meanwhile, add 1 tablespoon olive oil to a frying pan and set over a high heat. Add the sweetcorn, and cook for about 4 minutes until golden. Transfer the sweetcorn to a bowl and add the coriander, tomato, kidney beans, and juice of 1 lime. Season with salt and freshly ground black pepper, mix well, then set aside.

4 In a small bowl combine the juice of 1 lime with the chipotle paste and honey. Set aside.

5 Add the remaining 1 tablespoon olive oil to the pan the sweetcorn was cooked in, then set over a high heat. Once hot, add the steak pieces and cook for about 4 minutes, turning, until golden in colour. Add the chipotle sauce and cook briefly – just until the sauce coats the steak and looks glossy – then set aside.

6 Divide the steak among four bowls, and add the sweetcorn salsa, sweet potatoes, avocados, and lettuce. Squeeze over the juice from the remaining lime, and serve.

Swap it: This would also work with halloumi or tofu instead of steak.

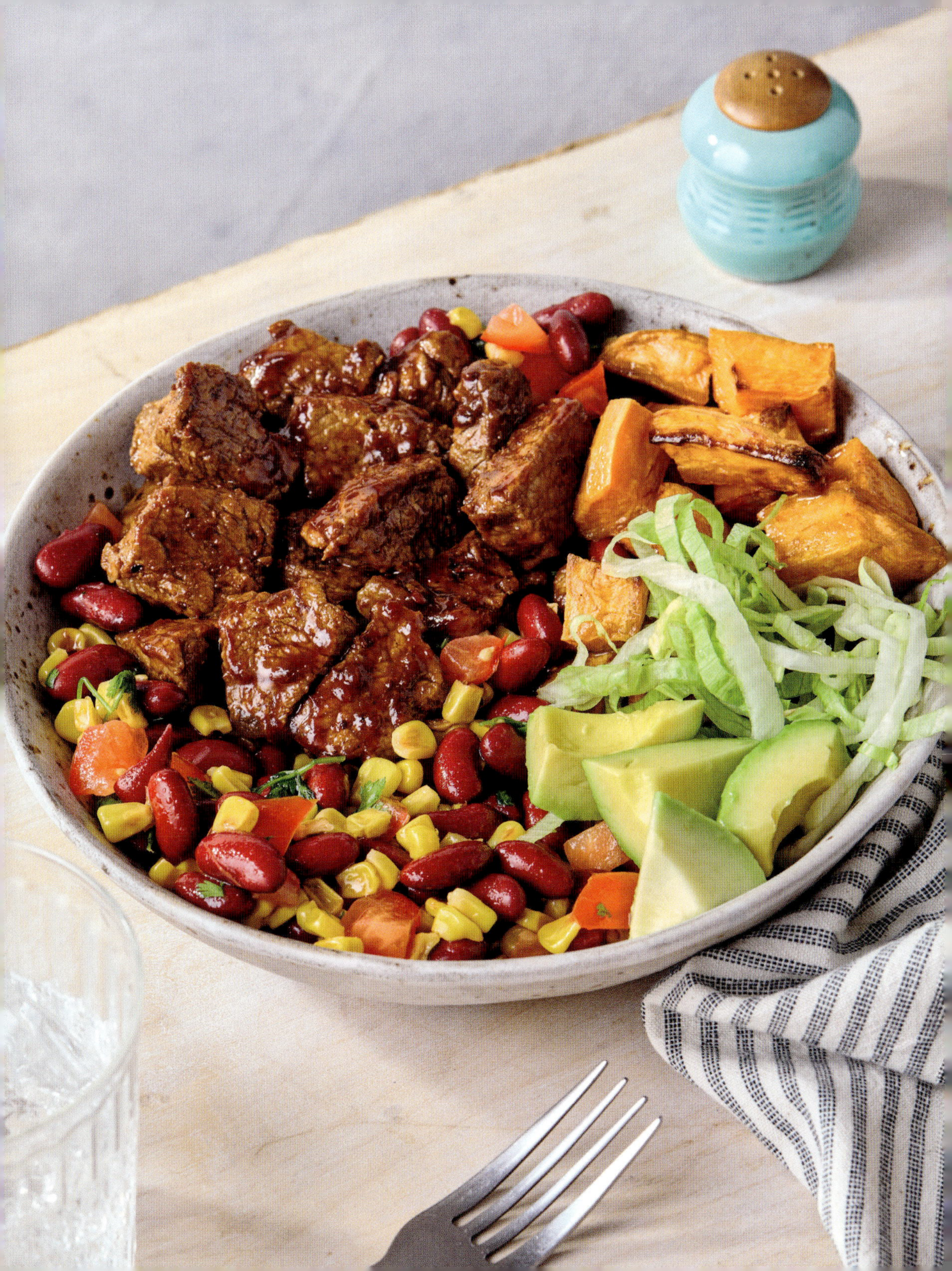

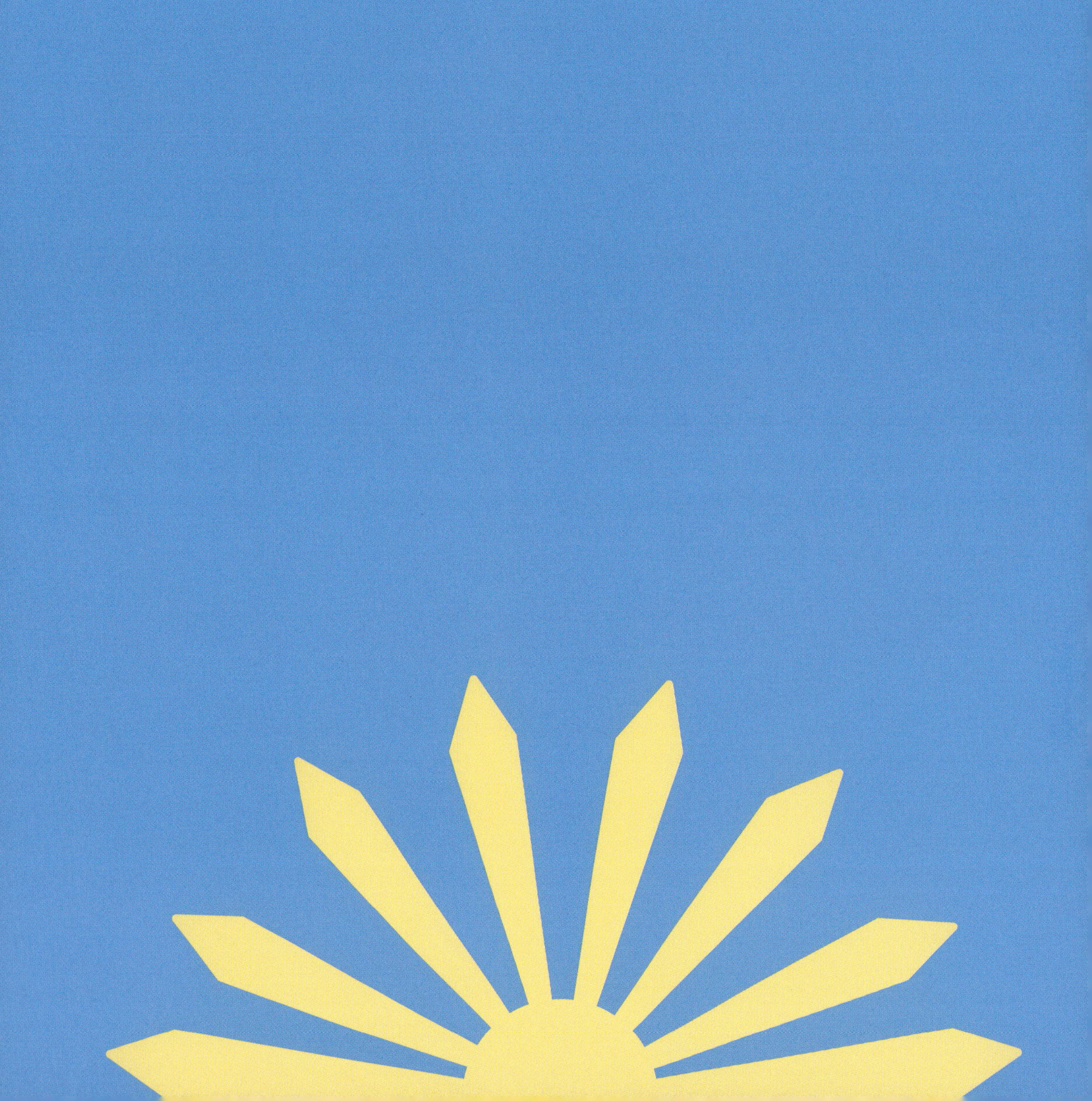

Midweek Dinners

Having some quick-and-easy midweek dinner ideas up your sleeve is a game changer. These recipes are so simple and quick to prepare, so you can still make it to the gym after a long day. From stir-fries and steamed fish to burgers and steaks, you'll find yourself coming back to these recipes again and again as part of your weekly routine.

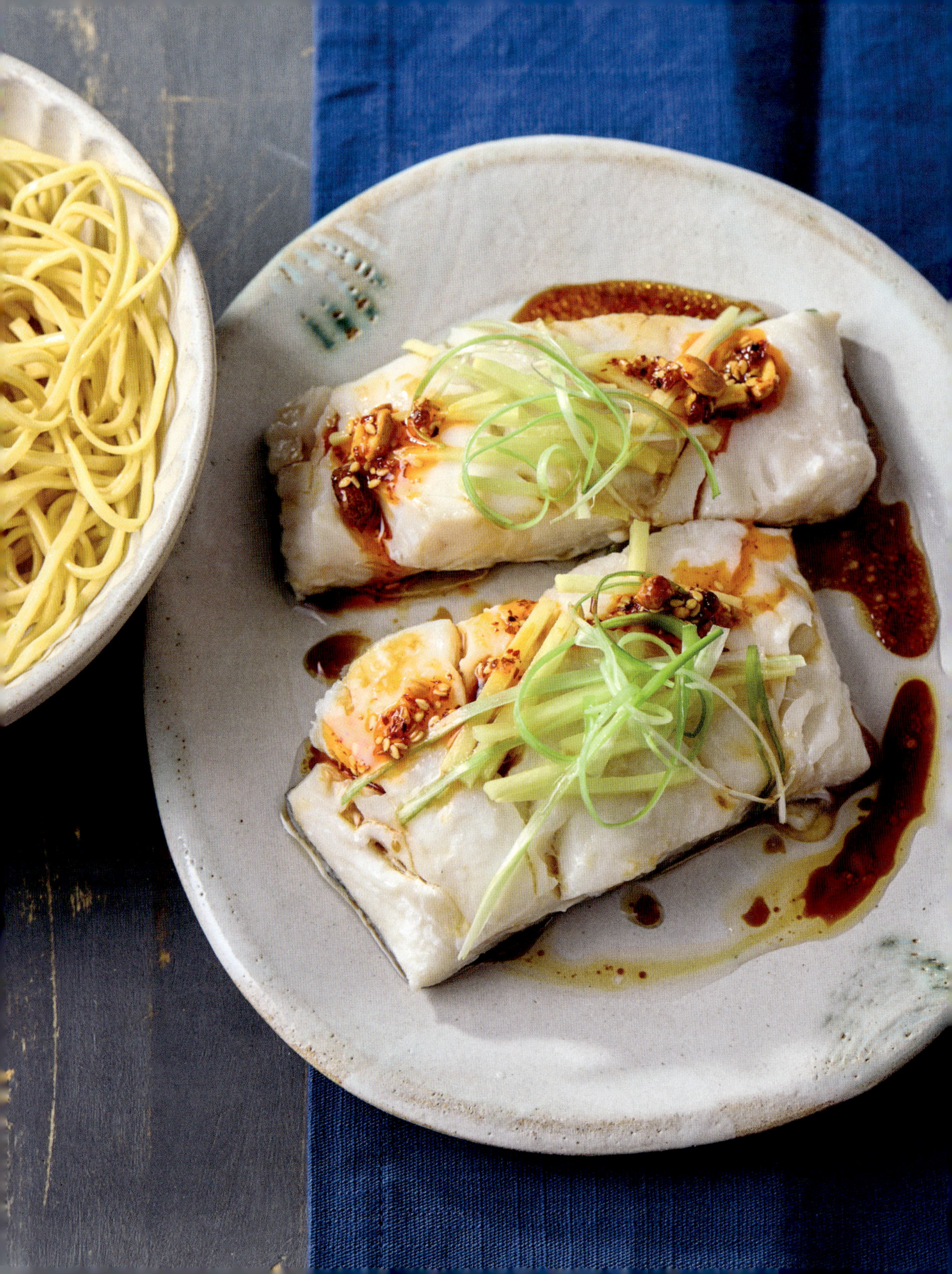

Soy Steamed Cod

Protein per serving: 41g **Kcals per serving: 633**

Serves 2

Prep + cook time: 20 minutes

2 large pieces of cod
5cm (2in) piece of ginger
4 spring onions
2 tbsp soy sauce
1 tbsp sesame oil
½ tsp caster sugar
1 tbsp crispy chilli oil
2 tbsp vegetable oil
160g (6oz) egg noodles
salt

To serve:
sesame seeds

Cod is a great source of low-fat high-quality protein.

1 Season the cod with some salt and set aside.

2 Fill a large saucepan (with a tight-fitting lid) one-quarter full with water, then set a steamer basket inside, making sure the basket does not touch the water. Set over a medium-high heat.

3 Slice half of the ginger into big slices, then cut half the spring onions into rough pieces. Place the spring onions and ginger onto a heatproof plate, and arrange the cod on top. Add the plate to the steamer basket, cover the pan with a tight-fitting lid, and cook for 12 minutes until cooked through.

4 Thinly slice the remaining spring onions. Cut the remaining ginger into matchsticks. Set aside.

5 In a small bowl, combine the soy sauce, sesame oil, sugar, crispy chilli oil, and 2 tablespoons water.

6 Once the fish is cooked, remove from the basket and pour away the water sitting on the plate. Pour the sauce over the fish and top with the finely chopped spring onion and matchstick ginger.

7 Cook the noodles according to the packet instructions and set aside. To a small saucepan, add the vegetable oil and set over a high heat. Once smoking, pour the oil over the spring onion and ginger on the fish. Sprinkle the sesame seeds over the fish and serve with the noodles.

Swap it: This would also work well with sea bass.

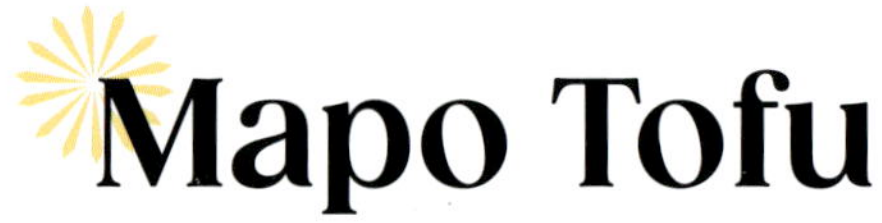

Mapo Tofu

Protein per serving: 35g **Kcals per serving: 751**

Serves 4

Prep + cook time: 15 minutes

- 1 tbsp vegetable or sunflower oil
- 200g (7oz) pork mince
- 2 cloves of garlic, crushed
- 2cm (¾in) piece of ginger, finely chopped
- ½ onion, finely chopped
- 2 tbsp white miso paste
- 1 tbsp soy sauce
- 1 tbsp oyster sauce
- ½ tbsp sesame oil
- ½ tbsp gochujang
- 1 tbsp soft light brown sugar
- 350g (12oz) firm silken tofu, cut into 2cm (¾in) cubes
- 2 x 250g (9oz) pouches of microwaveable basmati rice

To serve:

- sesame seeds
- finely chopped spring onion

1 Set a frying pan or wok over a medium-high heat, then add the oil. Once hot, add the pork mince, garlic, ginger, and onion, and cook for 5 minutes until golden.

2 Meanwhile, to a small bowl, add the miso paste, soy, oyster sauce, sesame oil, gochujang, and brown sugar. Mix well, then add into the pan, along with the tofu. Cook for a further 2 minutes until the tofu is warmed through, and then mix everything together, being careful not to break the tofu up.

3 Heat the rice in the microwave according to the packet instructions.

4 Serve the mince, tofu, and rice topped with sesame seeds and chopped spring onion.

Swap it: To make this veggie, just leave out the pork mince and oyster sauce.

Pork mince and tofu combine to offer a balance of complete proteins, iron, and calcium in this nutrient-dense and flavourful meal.

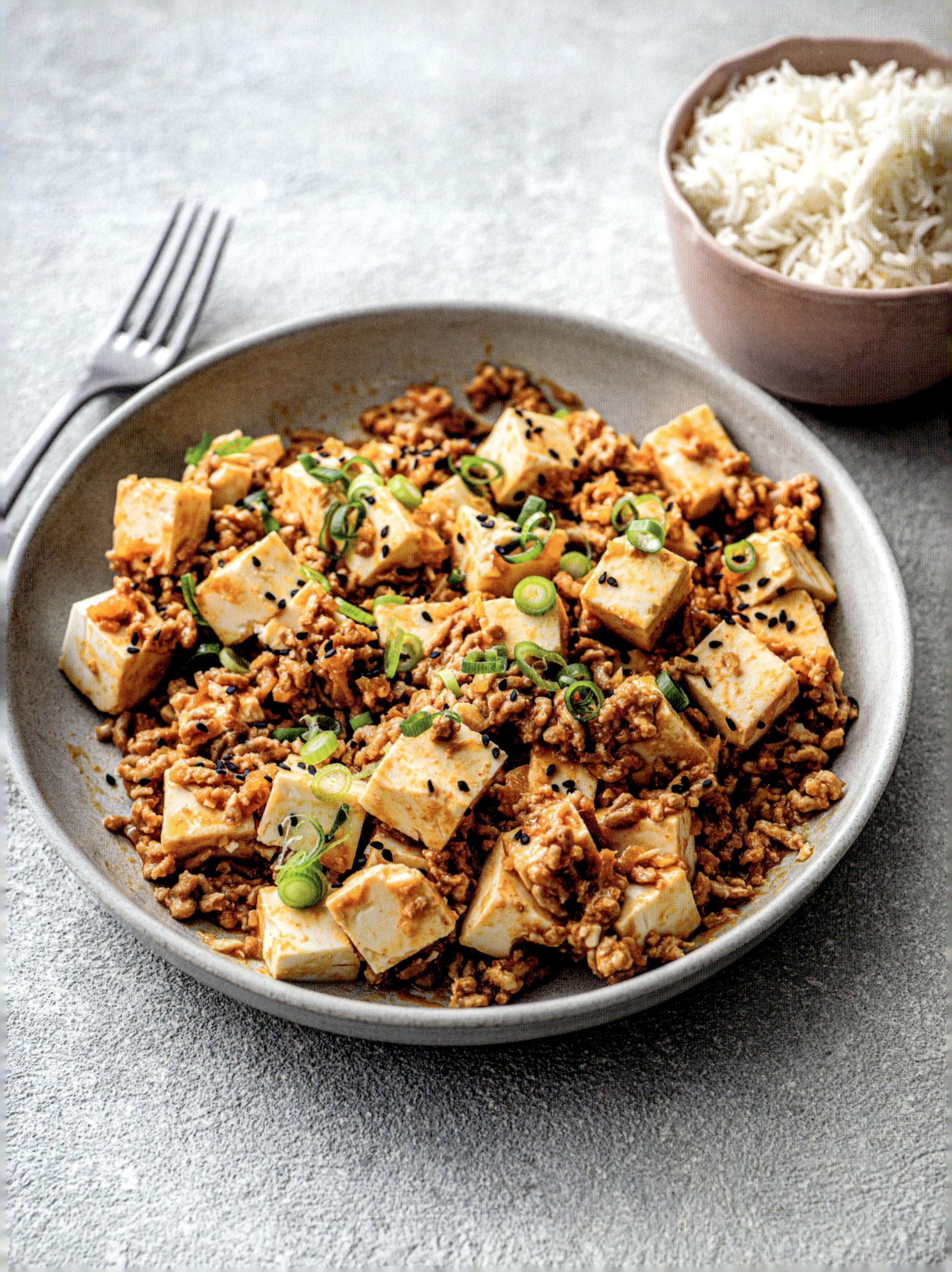

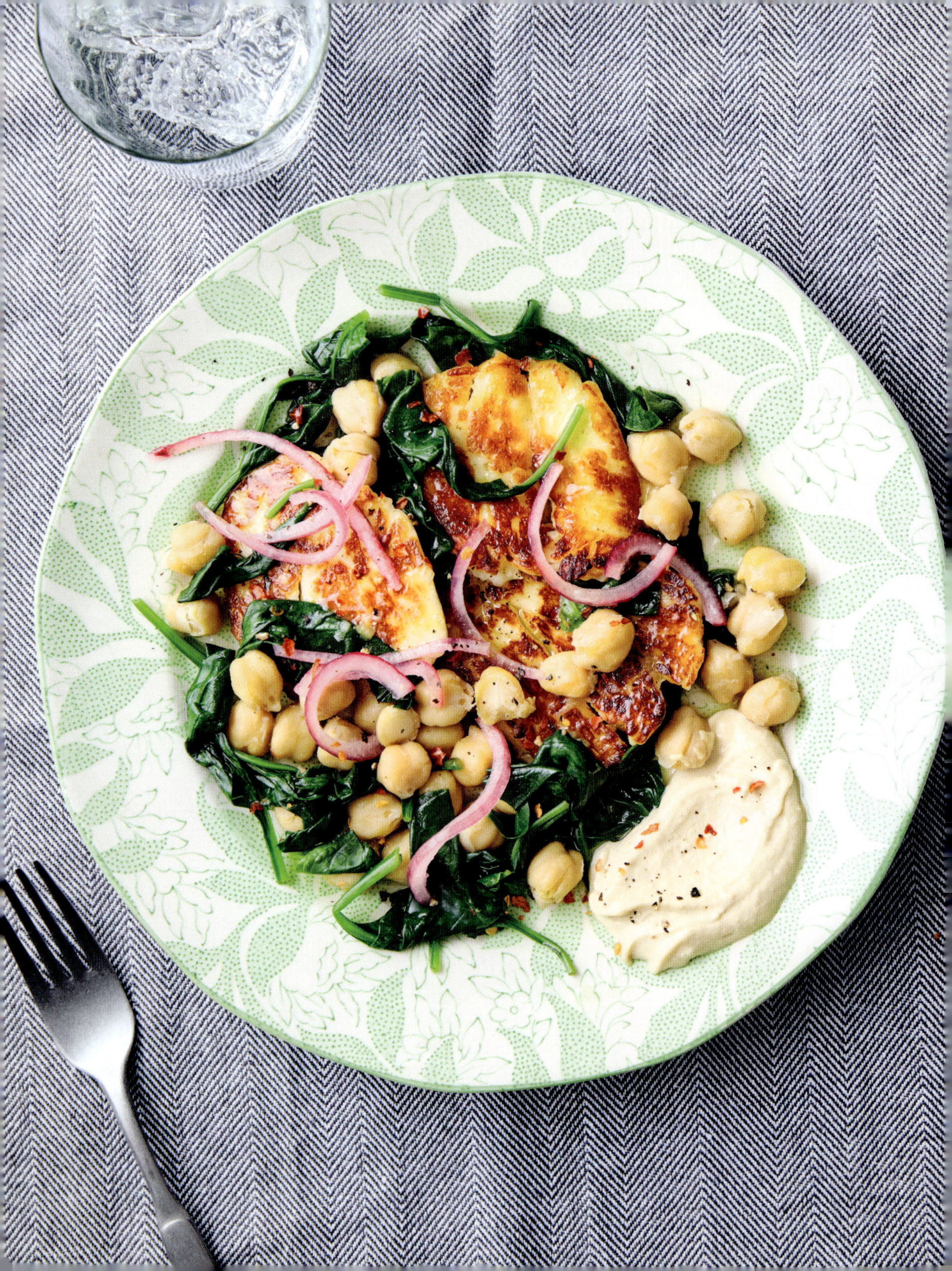

Halloumi with Chickpeas and Spinach

Protein per serving: 36g **Kcals per serving: 543**

Serves 4

Prep + cook time: 10 minutes

- ½ red onion, thinly sliced
- juice of 3 lemons
- 1 tbsp extra virgin olive oil
- 2 x 225g (8oz) packs of halloumi, cut into 3cm (1¼in) slices
- 400g (14oz) can of chickpeas, drained and rinsed
- 2 cloves of garlic, crushed
- 1 tbsp honey
- 200g (7oz) spinach
- pinch of chilli flakes
- salt and freshly ground black pepper

To serve (optional):

- 4 wholemeal pitta breads
- 200g (7oz) hummus

1 To a small bowl, add the red onion, the juice of 1 lemon, and a pinch of salt, then scrunch together with your hands and set aside.

2 Add the olive oil to a large high-sided frying pan with a lid, and set over a medium heat. Once hot, add the halloumi slices and cook for about 5 minutes, turning halfway, until golden in colour.

3 Lower the heat, then add the chickpeas, garlic, honey, spinach, and remaining juice from 2 lemons. Put the lid on, and cook until the spinach has slightly wilted.

4 Season with salt and freshly ground black pepper, top with the pickled onion, and sprinkle over the chilli flakes. Serve with pitta breads and hummus on the side, if liked.

Swap it: To make this vegan, use a vegan cheese alternative and swap the honey for maple syrup.

This dish is rich in protein, fibre, and iron, with spinach also providing folate, magnesium, and vitamin K.

Salmon Pasta with Peas

Protein per serving: 40g **Kcals per serving: 410**

Serves 4

Prep + cook time: 20 minutes

- 300g (10½oz) whole-wheat penne
- 100g (¾ cup) frozen peas
- 200g (scant 1 cup) Greek yogurt or crème fraîche
- 3 tbsp capers
- juice of 2 lemons
- 70g (2½oz) spinach
- 450g (1lb) hot smoked salmon
- handful of parsley, roughly chopped
- salt and freshly ground black pepper

1 Fill a large saucepan with water, season well with salt, and bring to the boil. Once boiling, add the pasta, and cook according to the packet instructions.

2 About 1 minute before the end of the cooking time, add the frozen peas. Reserve a cup of the starchy cooking water and drain the pasta.

3 Once drained, add the pasta and peas back into the pan. Add the yogurt or crème fraîche, capers, lemon juice, spinach, salmon, parsley, and a splash of the cooking water, and season with salt and freshly ground black pepper. Mix well then serve.

Tip: Use lentil pasta to up the protein even more.

Swap it: Tinned mackerel or tuna also works well here.

Whole-wheat pasta contains more protein than white varieties. Here it is paired perfectly with salmon and peas for a simple, high-protein midweek dinner.

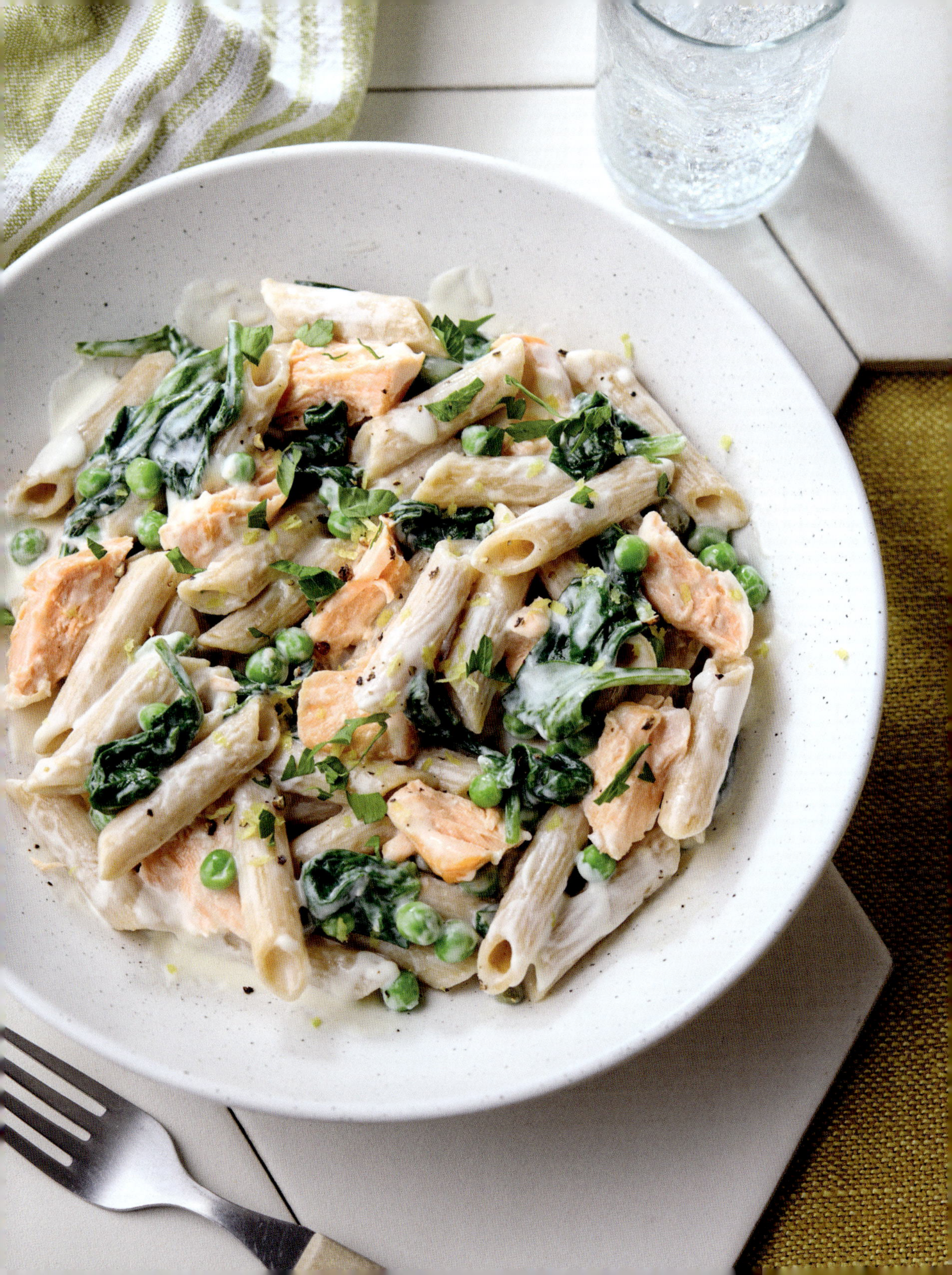

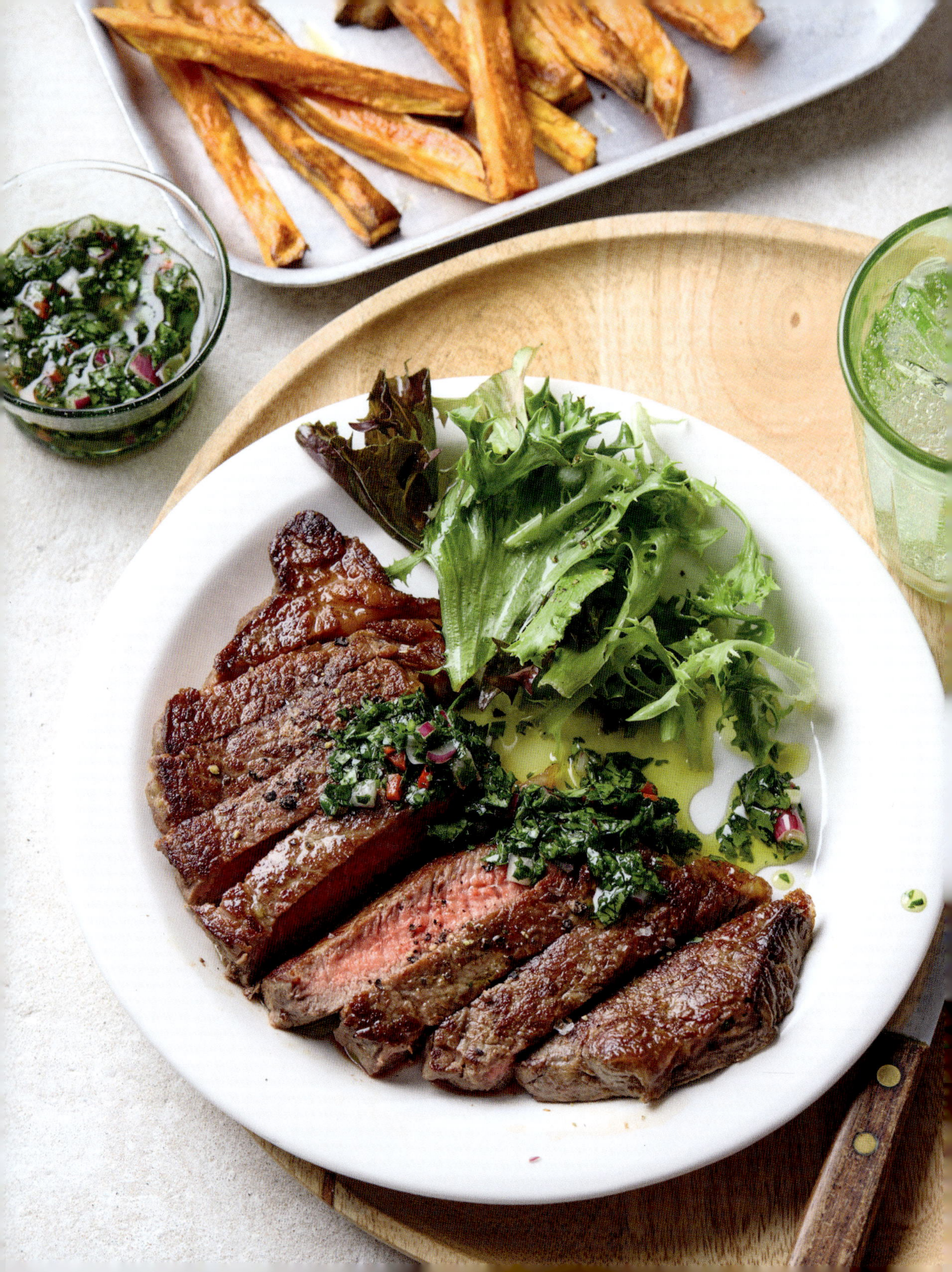

Steak with Chimichurri and Sweet Potato Fries

Protein per serving: 50g **Kcals per serving: 845**

Serves 2

Prep + cook time: 25 minutes

- 400g (14oz) sweet potatoes, peeled and cut into 2cm (¾in) batons
- ½ tsp cayenne pepper
- 2 tbsp vegetable oil
- large handful of parsley
- large handful of coriander
- ¼ red onion, finely chopped
- ½ red chilli, deseeded and finely chopped
- 1 tbsp red wine vinegar
- 65ml (4½ tbsp) extra virgin olive oil
- 2 x 200g (7oz) sirloin steaks
- salt and freshly ground black pepper

To serve:

salad leaves

Pairing sweet potato fries with protein-rich steak offers a nutrient-rich twist on a classic.

1 Preheat the oven to 200°C (180°C fan/400°F/Gas 6).

2 Put the sweet potato batons onto a large baking tray, sprinkle over the cayenne pepper, then drizzle over the oil and mix well. Spread the batons out on the tray, then cook for about 20 minutes, turning over halfway through, until cooked and crispy.

3 Meanwhile, to make the chimichurri, finely chop the parsley and coriander together, then combine with the red onion, chilli, red wine vinegar, and 50ml (3½ tablespoons) olive oil in a bowl. Season with salt and freshly ground black pepper, then mix well and set aside.

4 Drizzle the remaining olive oil over the steaks, then season well with salt and freshly ground black pepper.

5 Set a large frying pan over a high heat. Once hot, add the steaks and cook for about 2 minutes on each side for medium rare (or cook to your liking). Set aside to rest for 10 minutes.

6 Slice the steaks, then drizzle over the chimichurri. Serve the sweet potato fries on the side, along with some salad leaves.

Swap it: If you're short of time, simply cook some oven chips instead of sweet potato fries.

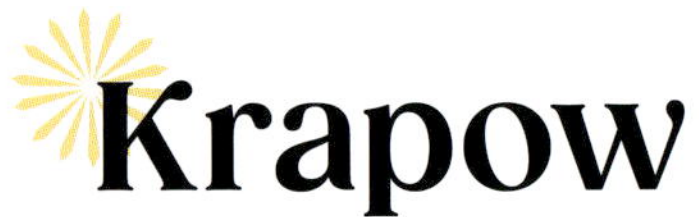

Krapow

Protein per serving: 48g **Kcals per serving: 541**

Serves 4

Prep + cook time: 15 minutes

- 2 tbsp vegetable oil
- 500g (1lb 2oz) chicken mince
- 1 onion, thinly sliced
- 100g (3½oz) green beans
- 1 red chilli, deseeded and finely chopped
- 2cm (¾in) piece of ginger, finely chopped
- 3 cloves of garlic, crushed
- 2 tbsp oyster sauce
- 1 tbsp fish sauce
- 2 tbsp soy sauce
- large handful of basil leaves
- 4 large eggs
- 2 x 250g (9oz) pouches of microwaveable basmati rice

1 Add 1 tablespoon oil to a large frying pan or wok, then set over a high heat. Once hot, add the chicken mince and cook for about 5 minutes, breaking it up with a wooden spoon, until golden in colour.

2 To the pan, add the onion, green beans, chilli, ginger, and garlic. Cook for a further 3 minutes until the vegetables have softened.

3 Add the oyster sauce, fish sauce, soy sauce, and basil. Mix well, turn off the heat, and set aside.

4 To a frying pan, add the remaining 1 tablespoon oil, then set over a medium heat. Crack in the eggs and cook for a few minutes until the whites of the eggs are set.

5 Meanwhile, microwave the rice pouches according to the packet instructions. Serve the chicken on top of the rice, and top each portion with a fried egg.

Swap it: Instead of chicken, you could use pork or turkey mince here.

The combination of chicken mince and eggs really boosts the protein content of this fragrant, Thai-inspired midweek dish.

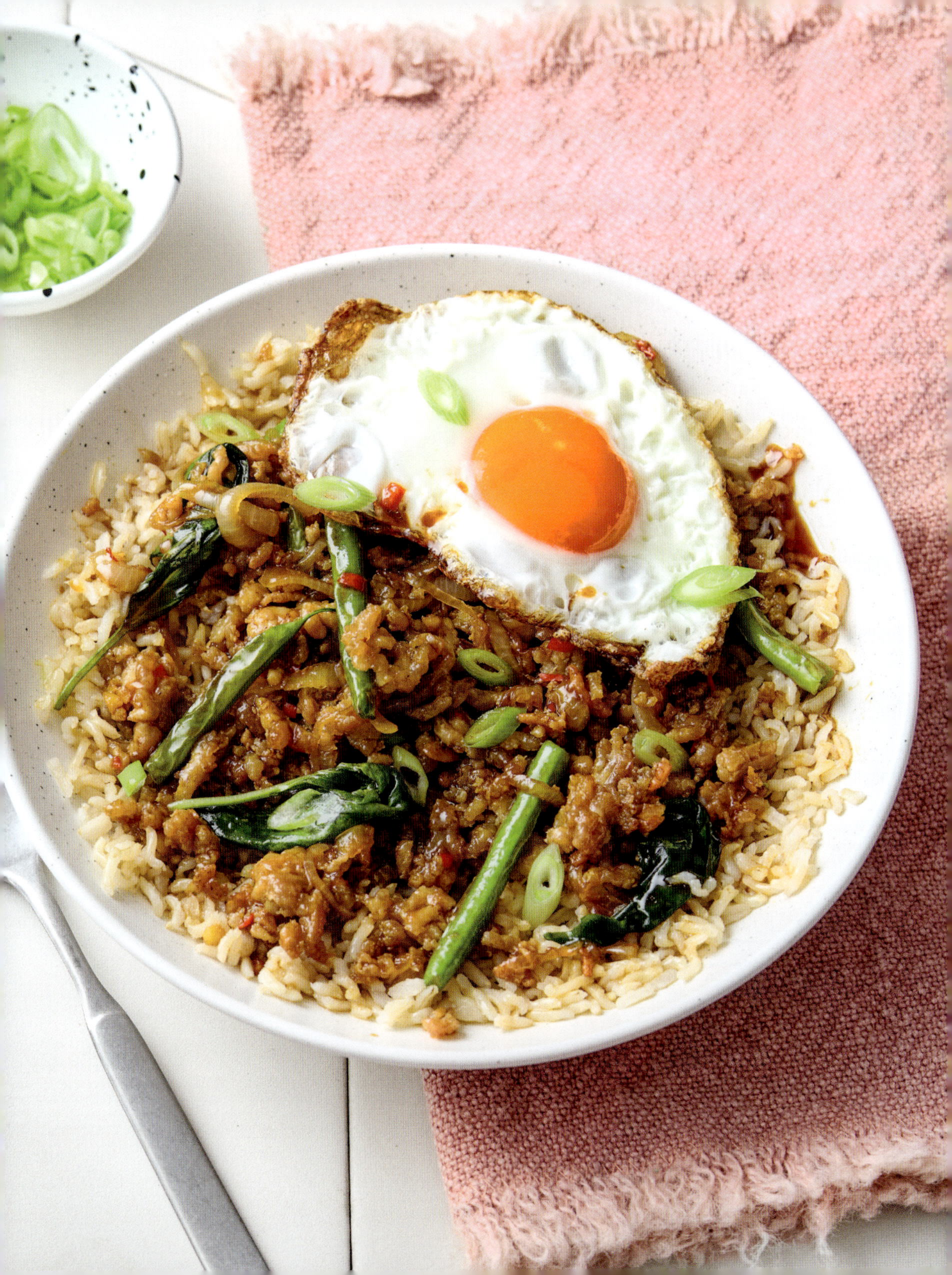

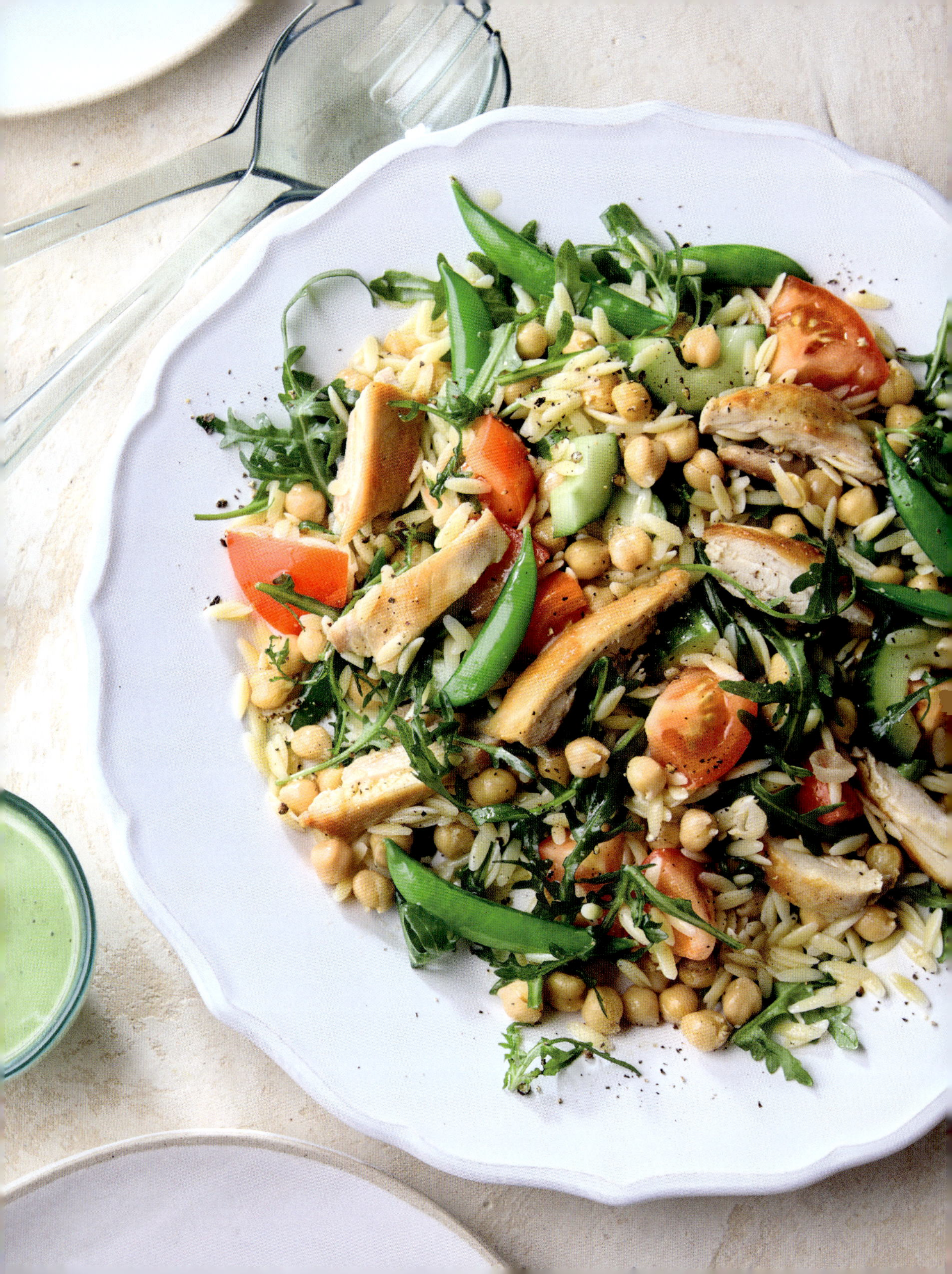

Chicken Orzo Salad

Protein per serving: 37g **Kcals per serving: 424**

Serves 4

Prep + cook time: 15 minutes

- 1 tbsp extra virgin olive oil
- 4 boneless, skinless chicken thighs
- 100g (3½oz) orzo
- 100g (3½oz) sugar snap peas
- 100g (scant ½ cup) Greek yogurt
- handful of basil leaves
- handful of parsley leaves
- 70g (2½oz) rocket
- juice of 1 lemon
- 2 tomatoes, cut into chunks
- ¼ cucumber, cut into chunks
- 400g (14oz) can of chickpeas, drained and rinsed
- salt and freshly ground black pepper

1 Drizzle the olive oil over the chicken. Set a griddle pan over a high heat and fry the chicken for about 10 minutes, turning halfway through, until cooked through and golden in colour. Cut into 3cm (1¼in) pieces, then set aside.

2 Meanwhile, fill a saucepan with water and bring to the boil. Once boiling, add the orzo and cook according to the packet instructions. About 2 minutes before the end of the cooking time, add in the sugar snap peas.

3 Meanwhile, to a blender add the yogurt, basil, parsley, a handful of the rocket, the lemon juice, and a pinch of salt. Blitz to make a dressing, then set aside.

4 Drain the orzo and peas, then add to a large bowl. Add the tomatoes, cucumber, chickpeas, chicken, and remaining rocket.

5 Drizzle the dressing into the bowl, then mix well and serve.

Tip: To make this veggie, omit the chicken and add feta and pumpkin seeds.

Using Greek yogurt here adds a creamy texture, and protein, calcium, and gut-friendly cultures.

Goan Fish Curry

Protein per serving: 33g **Kcals per serving: 472**

Serves 4

Prep + cook time: 25 minutes

- 4 large cod fillets, cut into 5cm (2in) chunks
- 1 tsp ground turmeric
- grated zest and juice of 1 lime
- 3 tbsp vegetable oil
- 1 onion, thinly sliced
- 3 large tomatoes, roughly chopped
- 3 tbsp Goan curry paste or other curry paste
- 400ml (14oz) can of coconut milk
- 2 x 250g (9oz) pouches of microwaveable basmati rice
- salt and freshly ground black pepper

To serve (optional):

- coriander leaves
- lime wedges

1 Put the cod pieces into a bowl and add the ground turmeric, lime zest and juice, and 1 tablespoon oil. Season with salt and freshly ground black pepper, then mix well and set aside.

2 Add the remaining 2 tablespoons oil to a saucepan set over a low-medium heat. Add the onion and fry for 5–10 minutes until softened.

3 Add the tomatoes and curry paste, then cook for a further 5 minutes until softened.

4 Add the coconut milk, along with a large pinch of salt and freshly ground black pepper, bring to the boil, then reduce the heat to low.

5 Blitz the sauce with a stick blender until smooth.

6 Add the cod pieces and cook over a gentle heat for about 5 minutes until the cod is cooked through.

7 Heat the rice pouch in the microwave according to the packet instructions.

8 Divide the rice among four bowls, top with the curry, and serve with coriander leaves and lime wedges, if liked.

Swap it: Other white fish or prawns would also work well here.

Cod is the hero here – providing lean protein and a natural source of iodine.

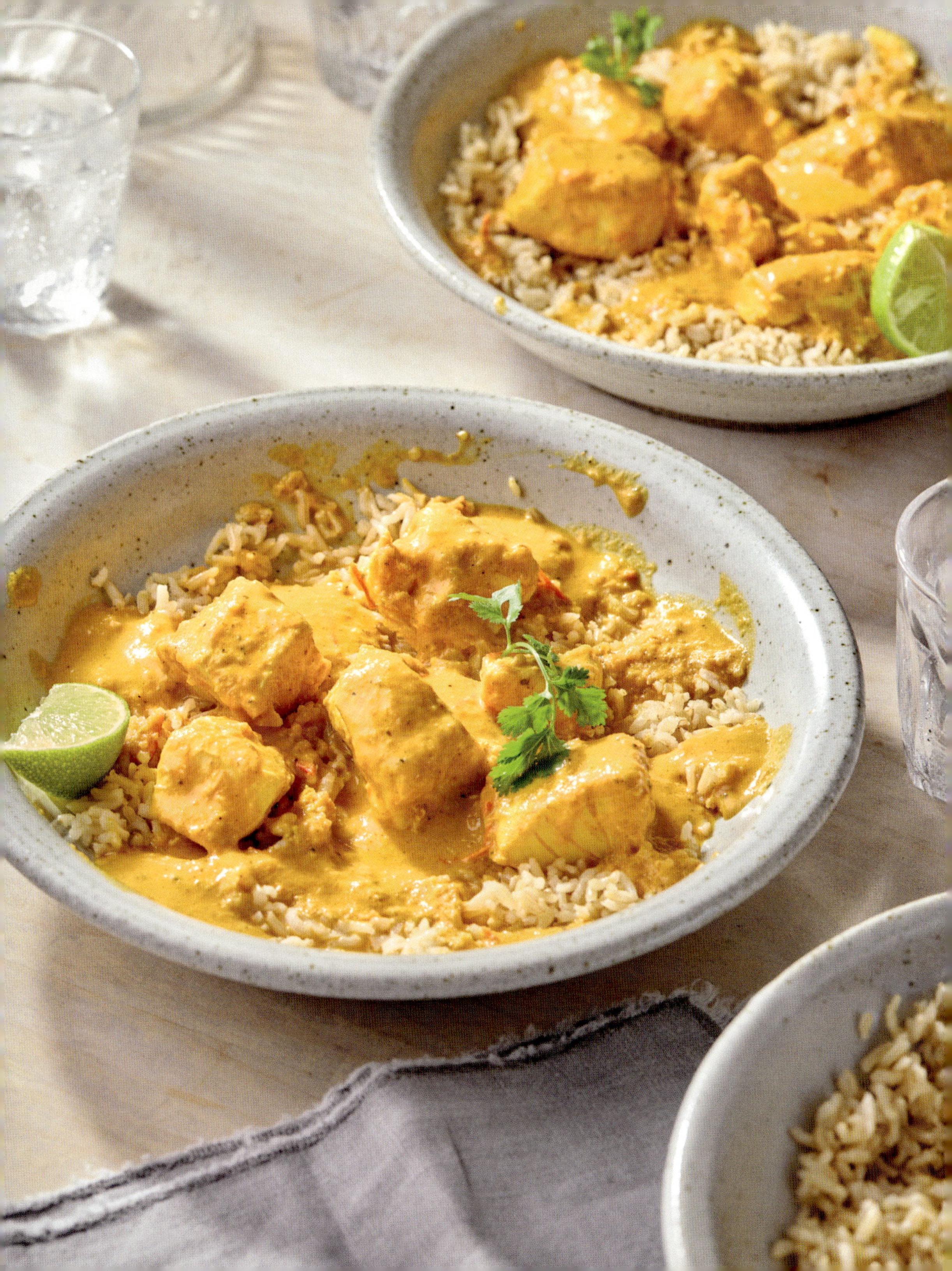

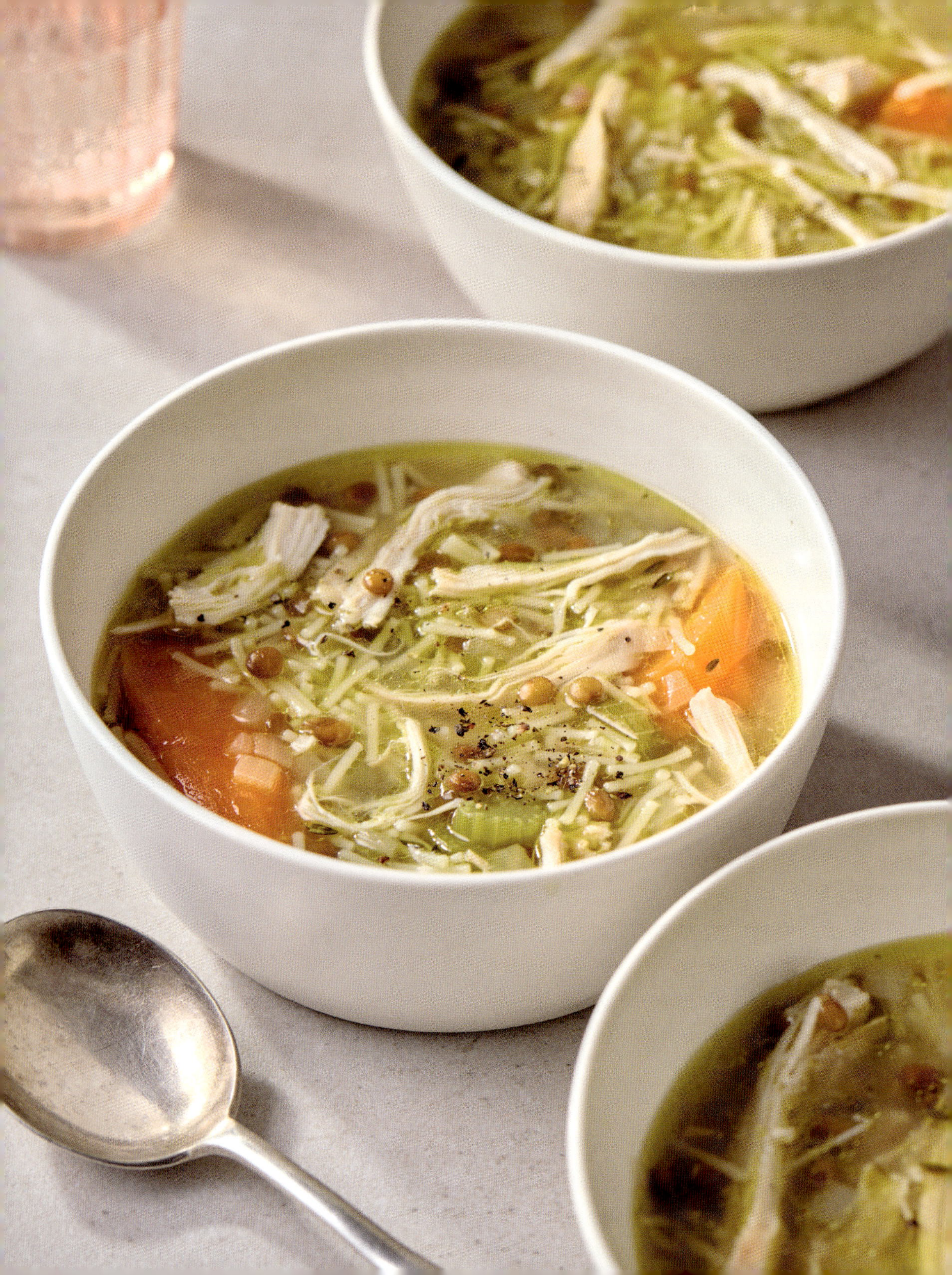

Slow Cooker Chicken and Green Lentil Soup

Protein per serving: 45g **Kcals per serving: 463**

Serves 4

Prep + cook time: 8 hours 30 minutes

- 2 cloves of garlic, crushed
- 2cm (¾in) piece of ginger, finely chopped
- 6 skinless chicken thighs
- 2 carrots, roughly chopped
- 1 onion, finely chopped
- 2 celery sticks, finely chopped
- 4 sprigs of thyme
- 2 bay leaves
- 2 litres (8½ cups) chicken stock
- 300g (10½oz) vermicelli noodles
- 400g (14oz) can of green lentils, drained and rinsed
- juice of 1 lemon
- salt and freshly ground black pepper

1 Set a slow cooker to low, then add in the garlic, ginger, chicken, carrots, onion, celery, thyme, bay leaves, and chicken stock. Cook on low for 8 hours.

2 Remove the chicken and shred it, discarding the bones. Add it back into the pot, along with the noodles and lentils, then cook for 15 minutes until the noodles are tender.

3 Add the lemon juice, then season with salt and freshly ground black pepper.

Keep it: This would freeze well for up to 3 months.

This comforting, nutrient-packed meal combines lean protein, iron, and fibre to support energy, fullness, and gut health.

Spring Salmon

Protein per serving: 44g **Kcals per serving: 712**

Serves 2

Prep + cook time: 30 minutes

- 400g (14oz) new potatoes, halved
- 2 salmon fillets
- 200g (7oz) asparagus, trimmed
- 150g (scant 1¼ cup) frozen peas
- 2 tbsp capers
- 1 lemon, thinly sliced
- 2 spring onions, thinly sliced
- 2 sprigs of thyme
- 50g (½ cup) pitted green olives
- 2 tbsp extra virgin olive oil
- 3 tbsp Greek yogurt
- 1 tsp Dijon mustard
- salt and freshly ground black pepper

1 Preheat the oven to 200°C (180°C fan/ 400°F/Gas 6).

2 Fill a saucepan with water and bring to the boil. Once boiling, add the potatoes and cook for 10 minutes.

3 Drain the potatoes and put onto a large piece of baking parchment. Top the potatoes with the salmon fillets, asparagus, peas, capers, lemon slices, spring onions, thyme, and olives. Drizzle over the olive oil, then season with salt and freshly ground black pepper.

4 Bring the two long edges of the baking parchment together and fold over several times to seal like a parcel, then bring the short edges up and fold over to seal it completely.

5 Put on a baking tray and cook for 15 minutes until the salmon is cooked through and the potatoes and vegetables are tender.

6 Meanwhile, add the yogurt and mustard to a small bowl, mix well, then set aside.

7 Serve the salmon parcel with the mustard yogurt on the side.

Swap it: You could easily leave out the potatoes from this recipe for a very simple supper. Serve with some seeded bread and a fresh green leaf salad.

This dish is rich in omega-3 fatty acids (EPA and DHA), which support heart, brain, and joint health. It is recommended to eat at least one portion of oily fish per week.

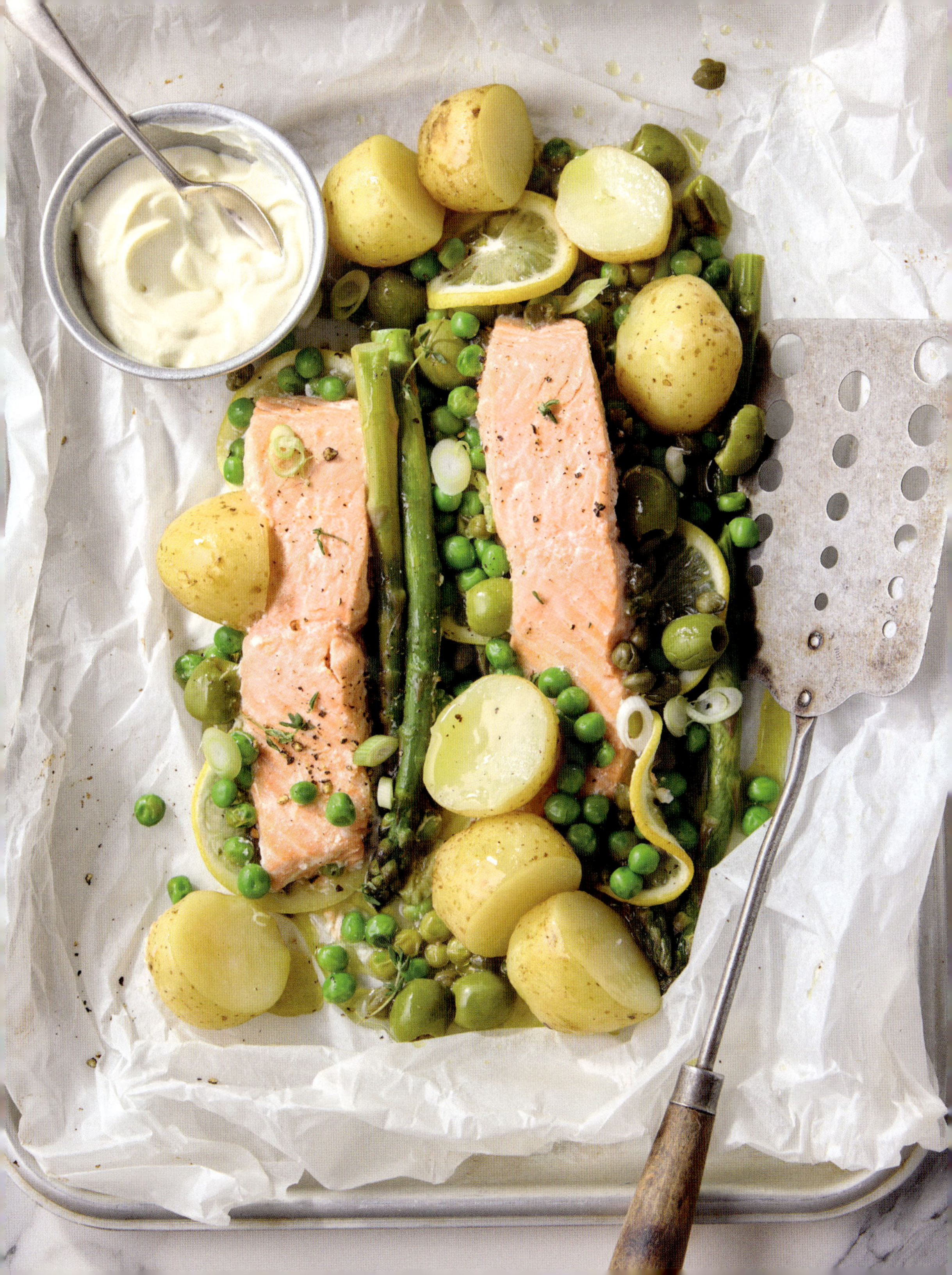

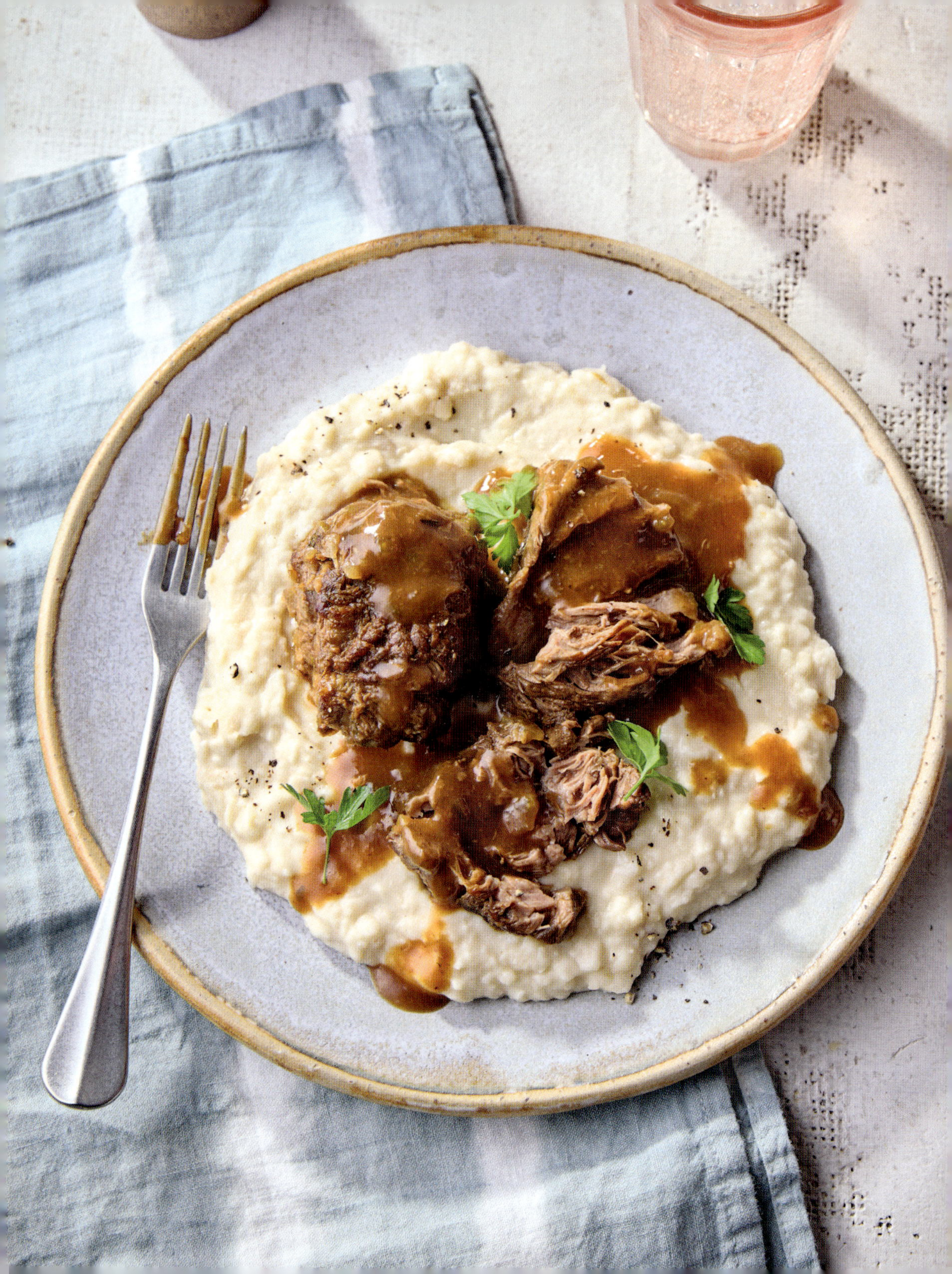

Slow Cooker Beef Stew with Butter Bean Mash

Protein per serving: 48g **Kcals per serving: 435**

Serves 6

Prep + cook time: 5–8 hours

- 1kg (2¼lb) braising beef, cut into 4cm (1½in) pieces
- 1 onion, sliced
- 3 cloves of garlic, crushed
- 2 carrots, roughly chopped
- 2 sticks of celery, finely chopped
- 2 tbsp tomato purée
- 2 bay leaves
- 500ml (2 cups) beef stock
- 1 tbsp extra virgin olive oil
- 2 x 400g (14oz) cans of butter beans, drained and rinsed
- juice of 1 lemon
- 1 tbsp wholegrain mustard
- salt and freshly ground black pepper

To serve (optional):
parsley leaves

1 To the slow cooker, add the beef, onion, 2 cloves of garlic, the carrots, celery, tomato purée, bay leaves, and beef stock. Cook on high for 5 hours, or low for 8 hours.

2 Shortly before the beef is ready, add the olive oil to a saucepan and set over a low-medium heat. Add the remaining garlic and cook for 30 seconds until fragrant.

3 Add in the butter beans and cook for a further 5 minutes, then add in the lemon juice and mustard. Season with salt and freshly ground black pepper, then mash with a masher or fork.

4 Serve the stew on top of the butter bean mash, topped with parsley, if liked.

Keep it: This stew will freeze well for up to 3 months.

This combination provides iron, protein, and fibre to support energy, muscle health, and fullness.

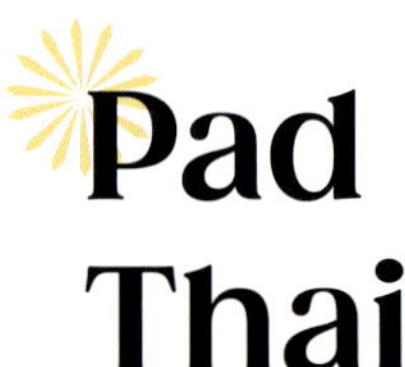

Pad Thai

Protein per serving: 31g **Kcals per serving: 588**

Serves 2

Prep + cook time: 15 minutes

- 1 tbsp vegetable oil
- 280g (10oz) block of extra-firm tofu, drained, pressed, and cut into 2cm (¾in) pieces
- 3 tbsp soy sauce
- 1 tbsp chilli garlic paste
- 1 tbsp maple syrup
- ½ tbsp fish sauce
- juice of 1 lime
- 250g (9oz) rice noodles
- 1 carrot, peeled into thin strips
- 200g (7oz) Tenderstem broccoli
- 2 tbsp peanuts, roughly chopped

To serve (optional):

- coriander leaves
- 1 red chilli, sliced

1 Add the oil to a large frying pan or wok, then set over a high heat. Once hot, add the tofu pieces and cook for about 4 minutes until golden and crispy on all sides.

2 Meanwhile, to a small bowl add the soy sauce, chilli garlic paste, maple syrup, fish sauce, and lime juice. Whisk together and set aside.

3 Fill and boil a kettle, then add the rice noodles to a large bowl. Cover the noodles with boiling water and let them sit for 2 minutes. Drain, run them under cold water, then set aside.

4 Add the carrot and broccoli to the tofu, then add in the sauce and cook for 2 minutes until the vegetables have softened.

5 Add the noodles to the pan and stir through the sauce until they are warm.

6 Divide the noodles between two bowls and sprinkle over the peanuts. Serve topped with coriander leaves and chilli slices, if you like.

Swap it: Prawns or chicken also work very well here.

This flavoursome dish serves up plant-based protein, calcium, and iron alongside crunchy, fibrous veggies.

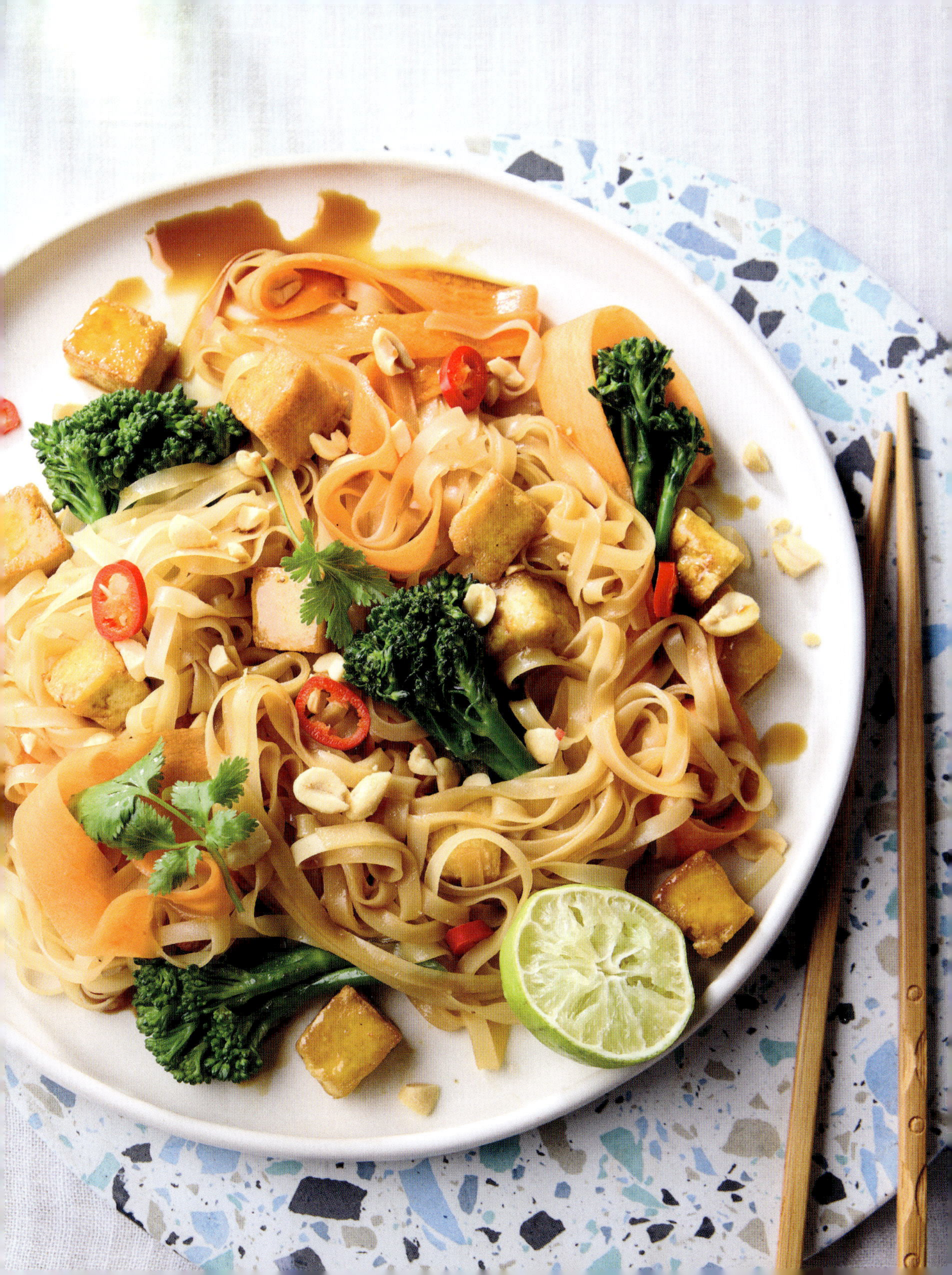

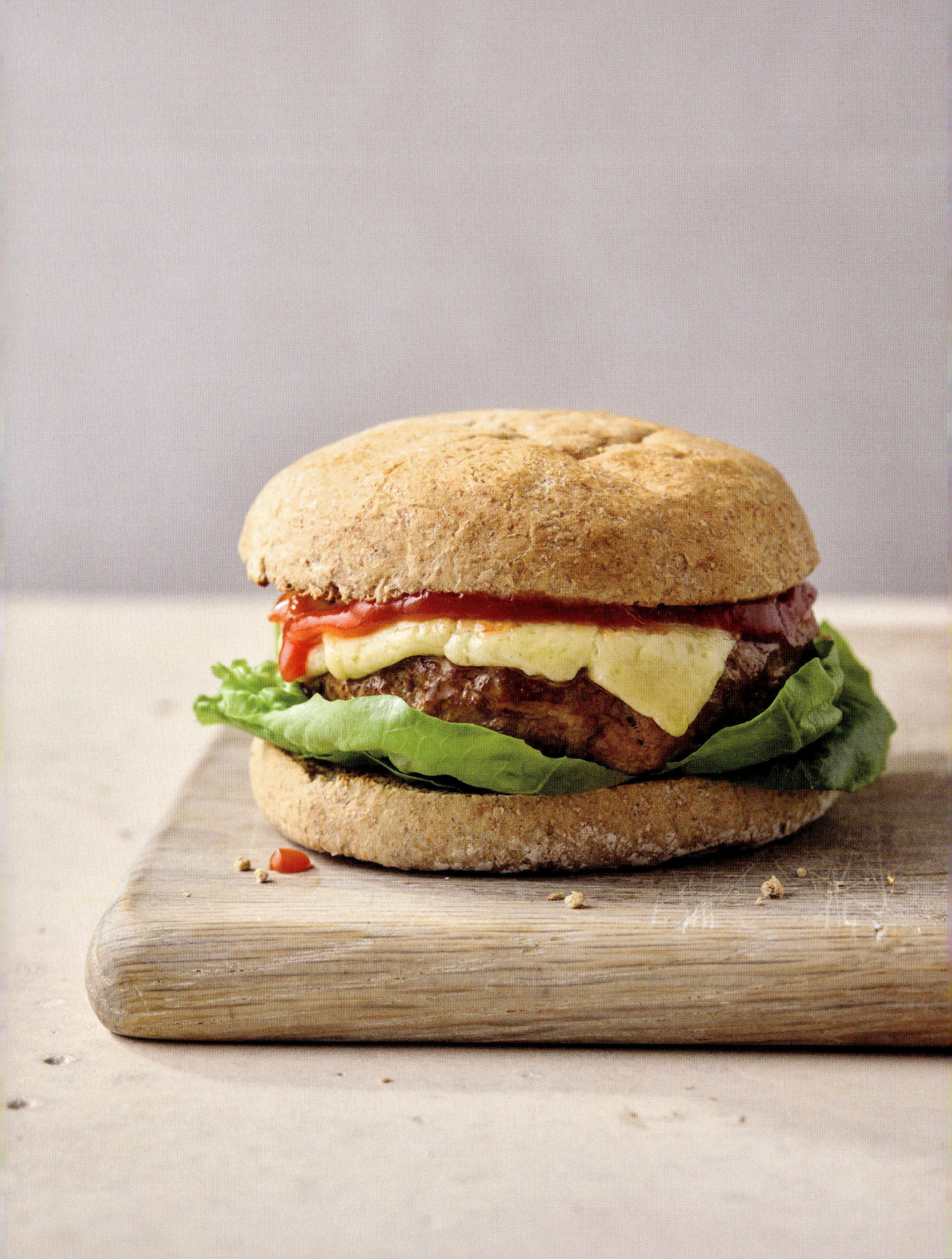

Turkey Burgers

Protein per serving: 37g **Kcals per serving: 428**

Serves 4

Prep + cook time: 20 minutes

450g (1lb) 4% fat turkey mince
1 red chilli, deseeded and finely chopped
handful of parsley, roughly chopped
splash of Worcestershire sauce
1 tbsp extra virgin olive oil
4 slices of Cheddar
4 burger or ciabatta buns
2 Little Gem lettuces, leaves separated
salt and freshly ground black pepper

To serve:
pickles
mayonnaise
ketchup

1 To a bowl, add the turkey mince, chilli, parsley, and a splash of Worcestershire sauce. Season well with salt and freshly ground black pepper, then shape the mixture into four patties, put them onto a tray, and set aside.

2 Add the olive oil to a large frying pan, then set over a high heat. Once hot, add the turkey patties and cook for 8 minutes, flipping over halfway through, until cooked through. Remove the patties from the pan, place a slice of cheese on each one, and set aside.

3 Cut the buns in half and add them to the pan, cut-side down, until toasted.

4 Arrange some lettuce on the bottom of the buns, top with the patties, pickles, mayo, and ketchup, followed by the tops of the buns.

Swap it: Beef or lamb mince also work well here.

Turkey mince is a lean source of high-quality protein, supporting muscle repair, fullness, and metabolic health.

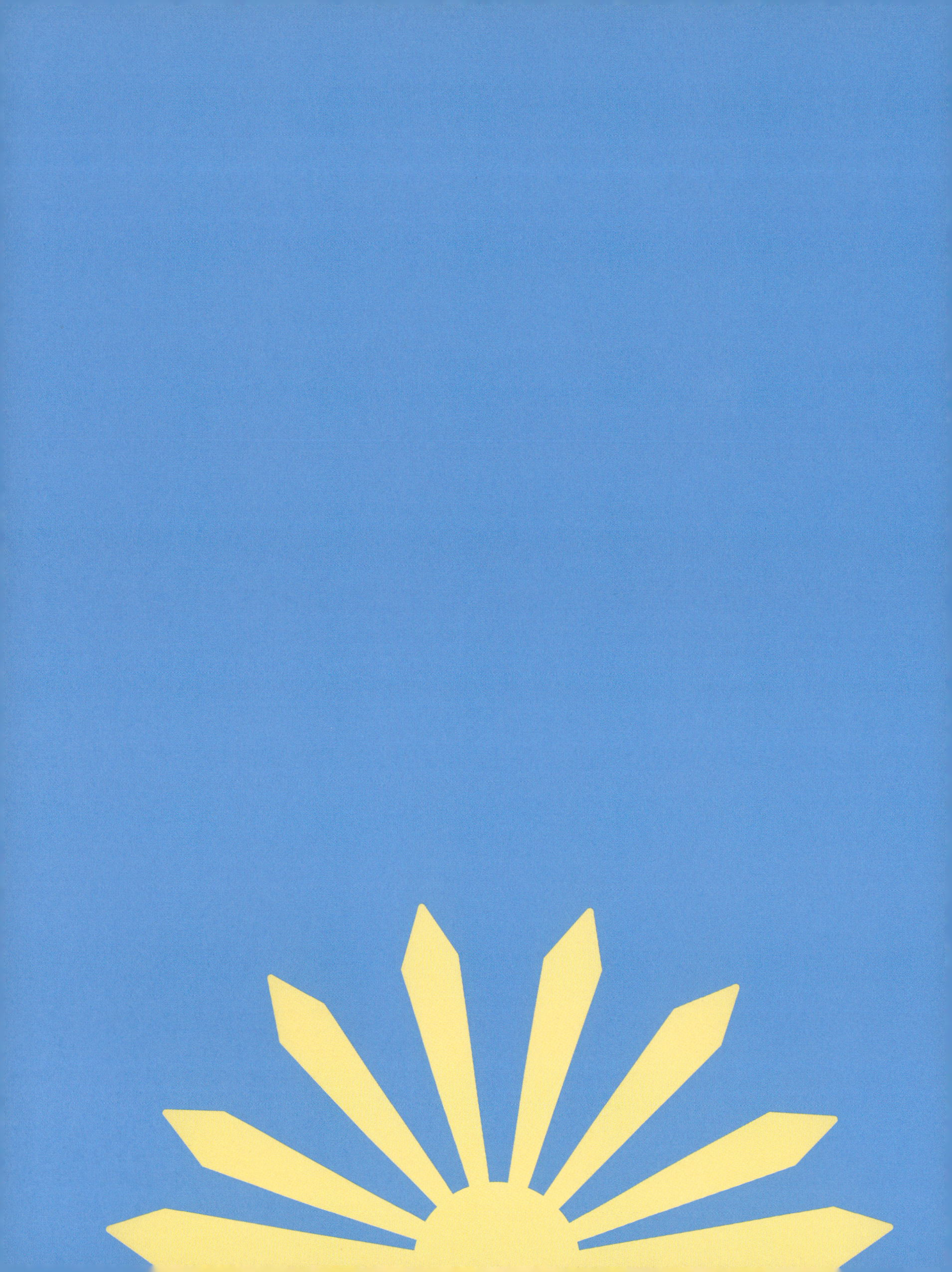

Batch Cooking & Meal Prep

Batch cooking and meal prep are essential when you're committed to maintaining a high-protein diet. Spend a rainy Sunday prepping these recipes and you can enjoy them throughout the week, or freeze them for later. Some of these recipes use a slow cooker to help you stay ahead of the game – your future self will thank you later!

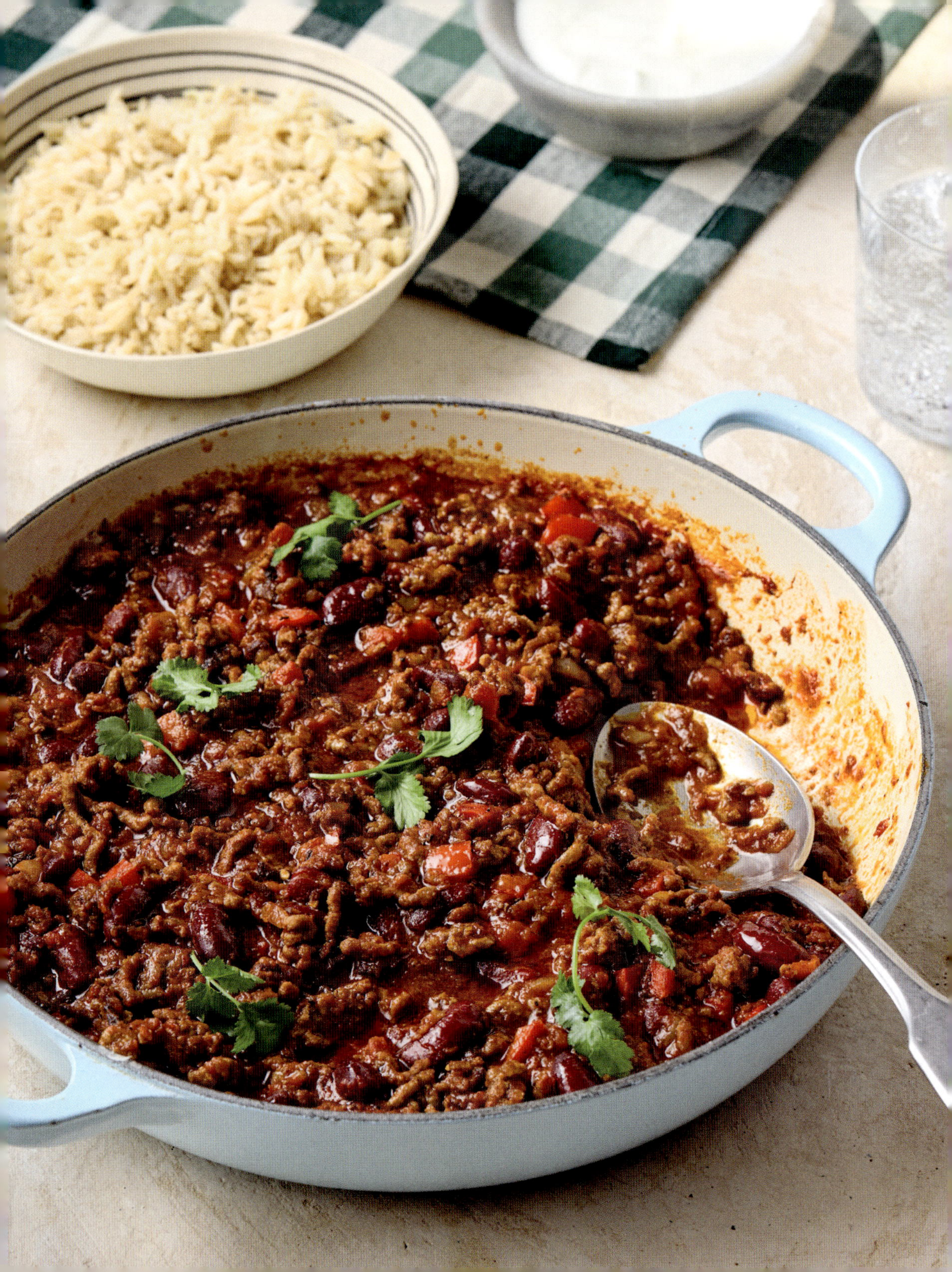

Chilli Con Carne

Protein per serving: 57g **Kcals per serving: 826**

Serves 4

Prep + cook time: 50 minutes

- 2 tbsp extra virgin olive oil
- 500g (1lb 2oz) 5% fat beef mince
- 1 onion, finely chopped
- 1 red pepper, finely chopped
- 2 cloves of garlic, crushed
- 1 tsp smoked paprika
- 1 tbsp dried oregano
- ½ tsp chilli powder
- 400g (14oz) can of chopped tomatoes
- 400g (14oz) can of kidney beans, drained and rinsed
- 300ml (1¼ cups) beef or chicken stock
- 2 x 250g pouches of microwaveable brown basmati rice
- salt and freshly ground black pepper

To serve (optional):

- natural yogurt
- coriander leaves

1 Add the olive oil to a large saucepan and set over a medium-high heat. Add the beef mince, then cook for about 5 minutes until the meat is browned.

2 Lower the heat, then add the onion, pepper, and garlic. Cook for another 10 minutes until the onion and pepper have softened.

3 Add the paprika, oregano, chilli powder, and a good pinch of salt and freshly ground black pepper. Cook for a further minute until fragrant.

4 Add the chopped tomatoes, kidney beans, and stock. Bring to the boil, then reduce the heat to low, cover, and simmer for 20–25 minutes until the sauce is thick and rich in colour.

5 Microwave the rice pouches according to the packet instructions, if using.

6 Check the chilli for seasoning, then serve with the rice, yogurt, and coriander, as liked.

Keep it: Store in the fridge for up to 4 days, or freeze for up to 4 months.

This brilliant high-protein staple is a flavourful way to load up on protein, iron, and fibre.

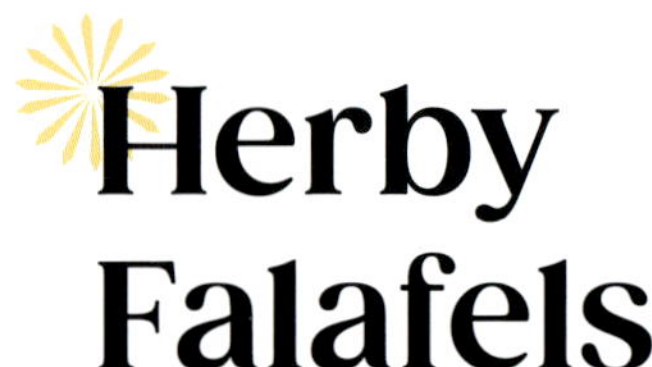

Herby Falafels

Protein per serving: 27g **Kcals per serving: 595**

Serves 2

Prep + cook time: 30 minutes

- 400g (14oz) can chickpeas, drained and rinsed
- 20g (⅔oz) parsley, roughly chopped
- 20g (⅔oz) coriander, roughly chopped
- 3 sprigs of mint, roughly chopped
- 1 clove of garlic, crushed
- ½ red onion, roughly chopped
- 1 tsp ground cumin
- 1 tsp za'atar
- grated zest of 1 lemon
- 2 tbsp sesame seeds
- salt and freshly ground black pepper
- vegetable or olive oil cooking spray

To serve:

- 2 pitta breads
- 2 tbsp hummus
- ½ romaine lettuce, shredded
- 1 tomato, sliced
- ¼ cucumber, sliced
- pickled green chillies

1 Preheat the oven to 200°C (180°C fan/ 400°F/Gas 6).

2 To a blender add the chickpeas, parsley, coriander, mint, garlic, onion, cumin, za'atar, and lemon zest. Season with salt and freshly ground black pepper, then pulse until the mixture comes together but still retains some texture.

3 Roll into 50g (1¾oz) balls, then roll in the sesame seeds. Arrange on a baking tray.

4 Spray the falafels generously with oil, then put into the oven and cook for 20 minutes until cooked through and golden in colour.

5 Serve with the pittas, hummus, lettuce, tomato, cucumber, and pickled green chillies.

Keep it: These will keep in the freezer for up to 3 months.

Chickpeas are rich in plant-based protein, fibre, and slow-release carbs, as well as iron, folate, and magnesium.

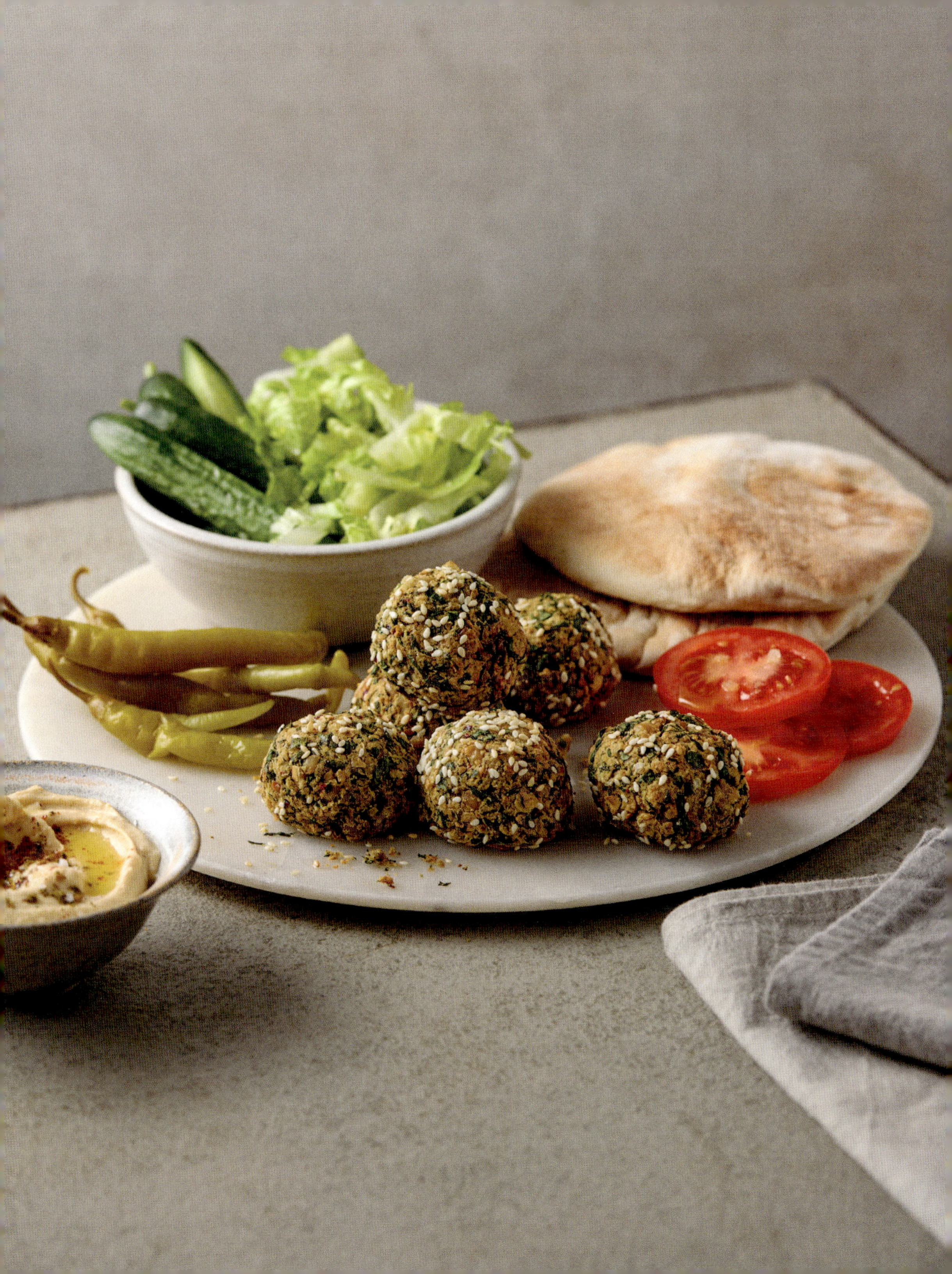

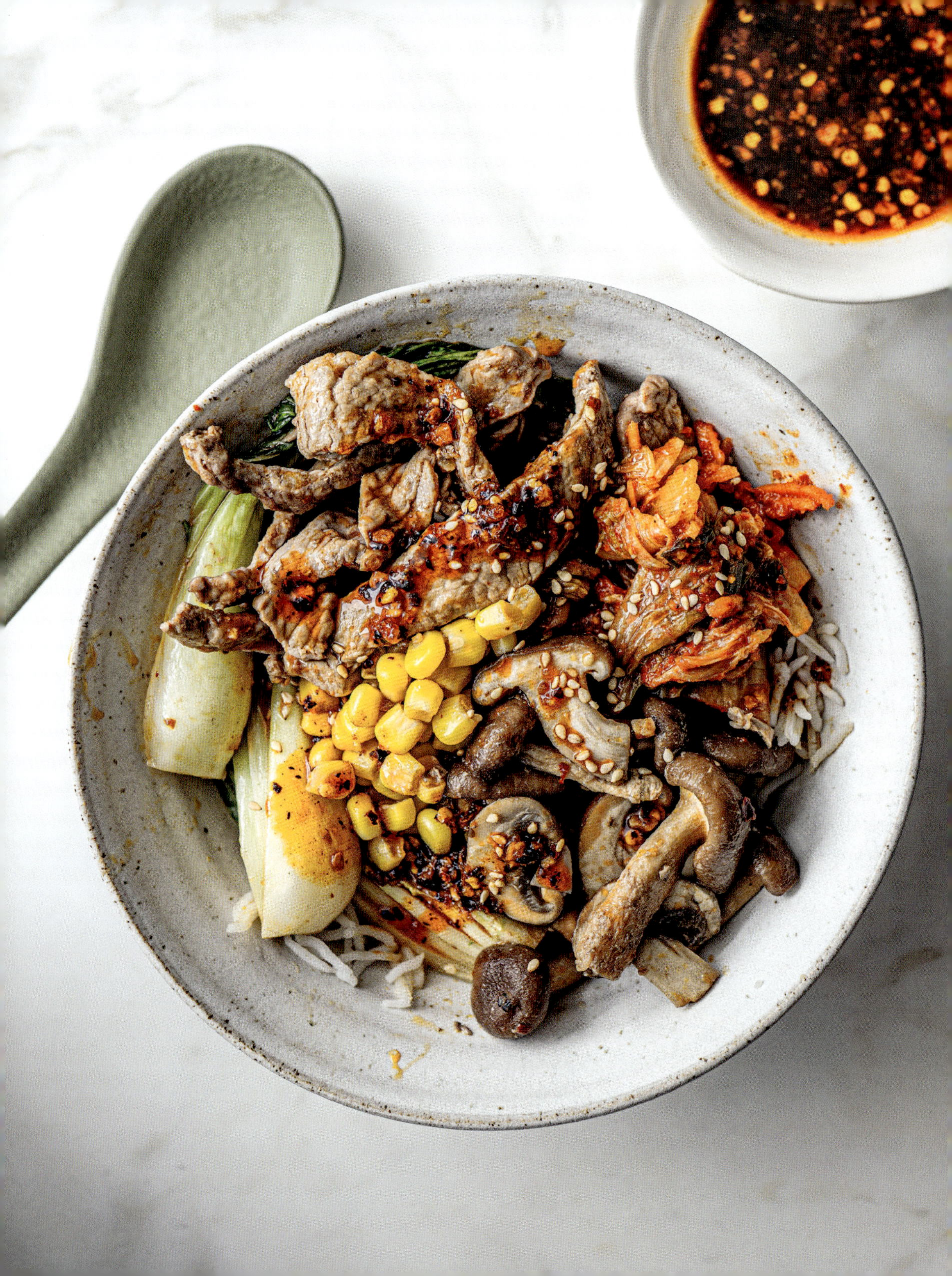

Steak and Kimchi with Dipping Sauce

Protein per serving: 40g **Kcals per serving: 611**

Serves 2

Prep + cook time: 15 minutes

- 50g (1¾oz) mushrooms, such as shiitake, enoki, or chestnut, thinly sliced
- 100g (⅔ cup) frozen sweetcorn
- 250g (9oz) pak choi, cut lengthways into quarters
- 250g (9oz) sirloin steak, fat removed, very thinly sliced
- 2 tbsp soy sauce
- 1 tbsp sesame oil
- 1 tsp crispy chilli oil
- 250g (9oz) pouch of microwaveable sticky rice
- 2 tbsp kimchi
- 1 tbsp sesame seeds

Dipping sauce:

- 2 tbsp soy sauce
- 1 tbsp rice wine vinegar
- 1 tsp crispy chilli oil
- 1 tsp mirin

1 Layer the ingredients in a saucepan for which you have a lid, one on top of the other: start with the mushrooms, then add the sweetcorn, pak choi, and steak.

2 Add the soy, sesame oil, and crispy chilli oil. Pour over 100ml (6½ tbsp) water.

3 Cover with a lid and bring to the boil. Once boiling, reduce the heat to low and cook for 5–10 minutes until the vegetables are tender and the steak is cooked through.

4 Meanwhile, in a small bowl, whisk together the dipping sauce ingredients. Set aside. Heat the rice according to the packet instructions. Set aside.

5 Top the steak with the kimchi and sesame seeds. Serve with rice, if using.

Swap it: To make this veggie, replace the steak with cubes of firm tofu.

Lean steak for protein, fibre-rich veg, and gut-loving kimchi – this dish is balanced, vibrant, and full of texture.

Red Lentil Soup

Protein per serving: 19g **Kcals per serving: 341**

Serves 4

Prep + cook time: 25 minutes

- 1 tbsp extra virgin olive oil, plus extra to serve
- 1 onion, finely chopped
- 3 cloves of garlic, roughly chopped
- 1 tbsp ground cumin
- 1 tbsp tomato purée
- 1 sweet potato, peeled and roughly chopped
- 1 large carrot, roughly chopped
- 200g (generous 1 cup) red lentils
- 1.6 litres (2¾ pints) vegetable stock
- juice of 2 lemons
- pinch of chilli flakes
- salt and freshly ground black pepper

1 Add the oil to a large saucepan with a lid, then set over a low-medium heat. Add the onion and garlic, and cook for about 5 minutes until softened.

2 Add the cumin and tomato purée to the pan and cook for 1 minute.

3 Add the sweet potato, carrot, lentils, and vegetable stock. Bring to the boil, lower the heat, then add the lid to the pan and cook for 15 minutes until the vegetables and lentils have softened.

4 Blitz with a stick blender until smooth, then season well with salt and freshly ground black pepper.

5 Divide among bowls, squeeze over the lemon juice, then top each portion with a pinch of chilli flakes and a drizzle of olive oil.

Serve it: Add a spoonful of cottage cheese to this soup when serving, if you like.

This is a simple way to get a plant-based protein boost, along with fibre, iron, and slow-release carbs.

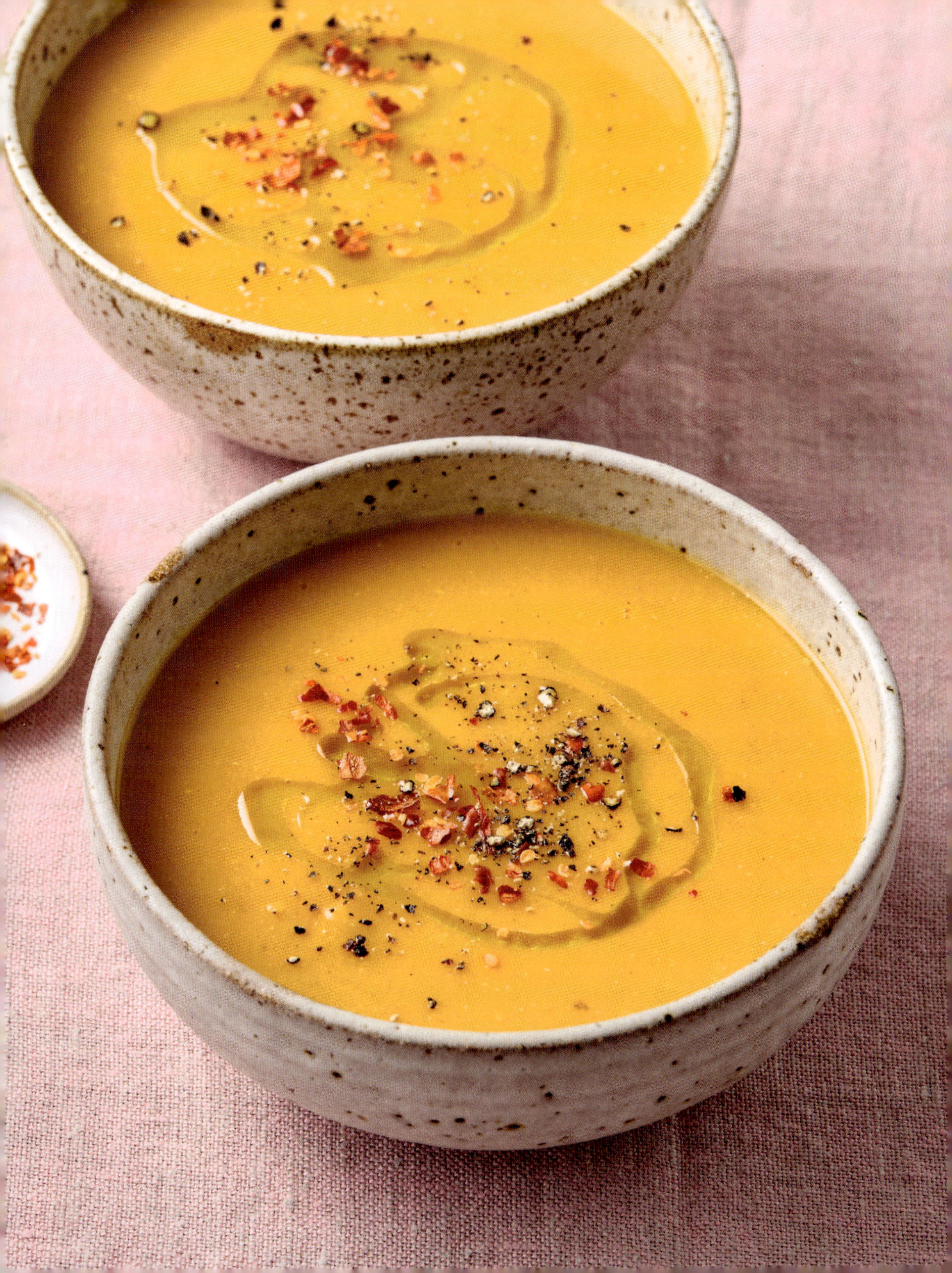

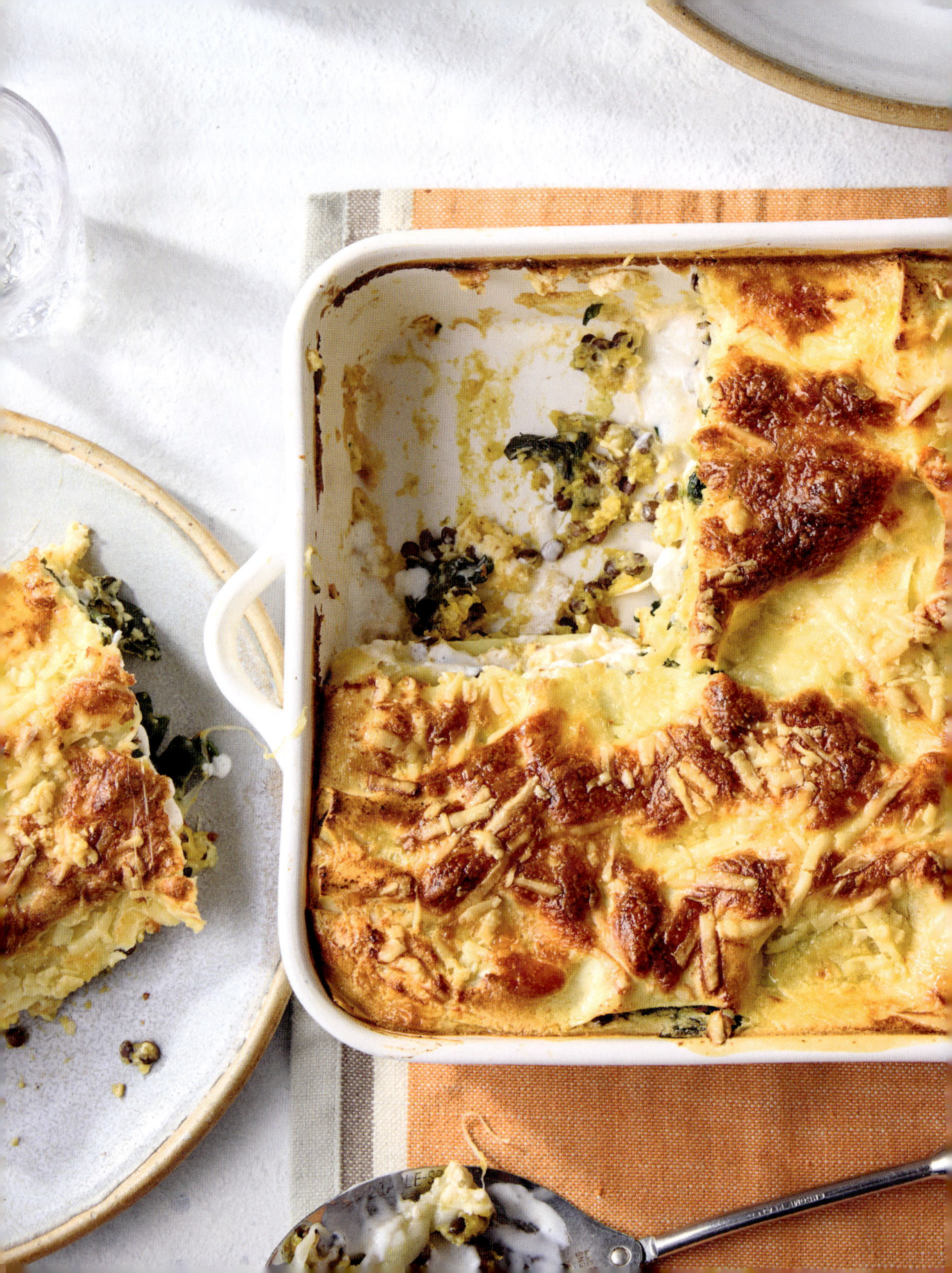

Butternut Squash Lasagne

Protein per serving: 44g **Kcals per serving: 770**

Serves 4

Prep + cook time: 1 hour 10 minutes

- 1 butternut squash, peeled and cut into chunks
- 4 cloves of garlic, bashed and kept in their skins
- 2 tbsp extra virgin olive oil
- 350g (1½ cups) cottage cheese
- 200g (scant 1 cup) Greek yogurt
- 2 large eggs
- pinch of nutmeg
- grated zest of 1 lemon
- 200g (7oz) spinach
- 250g (9oz) pouch of microwaveable green lentils
- 200g (2 cups) grated mozzarella
- 250g (9oz) fresh pasta sheets
- salt and freshly ground black pepper

Cottage cheese adds a creamy texture and a protein boost to this wholesome vegetarian dish.

1 Preheat the oven to 200°C (180°C fan/400°F/Gas 6).

2 Put the butternut squash and garlic onto a large baking tray. Drizzle over the olive oil, then season with salt and pepper. Roast for 20 minutes until the squash and garlic have softened.

3 Meanwhile, in a blender, blitz the cottage cheese, yogurt, eggs, nutmeg, lemon zest, and a pinch of salt until smooth. Transfer to a bowl and set aside.

4 Fill and boil a kettle, then add the spinach to a colander over the sink. Pour the boiling water over the spinach until wilted. Once cool enough to handle, squeeze the water out of the spinach, then roughly chop and set aside.

5 To a blender add the butternut squash, then squeeze the garlic out of its skin and add this into the blender. Blitz until smooth. Add the green lentils and stir through until combined.

6 In a medium baking dish, add a layer of the cottage cheese sauce, followed by a layer of the butternut squash filling. Top this with the spinach, mozzarella, and a pasta sheet. Repeat this until everything is used up, finishing with a layer of the cottage cheese mix and the mozzarella. Bake in the oven for 30–35 minutes until bubbling.

Keep it: This is a great meal prep dish. It will keep in the fridge once baked for up to 5 days.

Mango Chutney Chicken Sandwich Filling

Protein per serving: 44g **Kcals per serving: 470**

Serves 4

Prep time: 15 minutes

- 1 rotisserie-cooked chicken
- ½ red onion, finely chopped
- handful of chives, finely chopped
- 2 large tomatoes, deseeded and finely chopped
- 90g (⅓ cup) mango chutney
- juice of 1 lemon
- 80g (generous ⅓ cup) Greek yogurt
- 60g (¼ cup) mayonnaise
- salt and freshly ground black pepper

1 Shred the chicken and put it into a bowl.

2 Add the red onion, chives, tomatoes, mango chutney, lemon juice, Greek yogurt, and mayo. Season with salt and freshly ground black pepper, then mix well.

3 Cover and put into the fridge until ready to use.

Keep it: This will keep refrigerated for up to 5 days.

Serve it: This would be perfect in a wrap, sandwich, or toastie, or simply served with some green lettuce as a salad.

Lean protein is combined with a touch of sweetness and spice in a tasty filling that supports muscle health and satiety, and makes for an easy, high-protein lunch option.

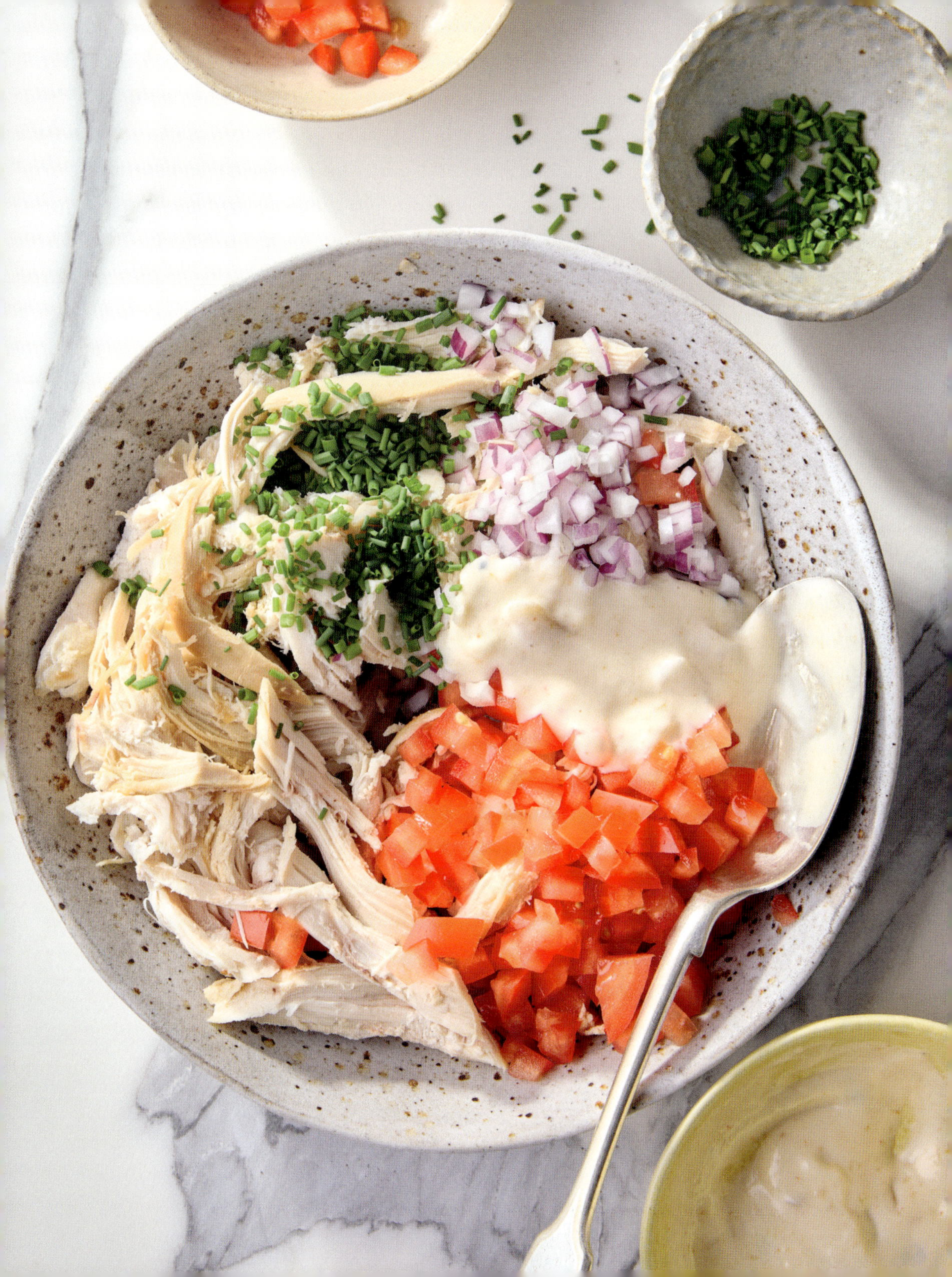

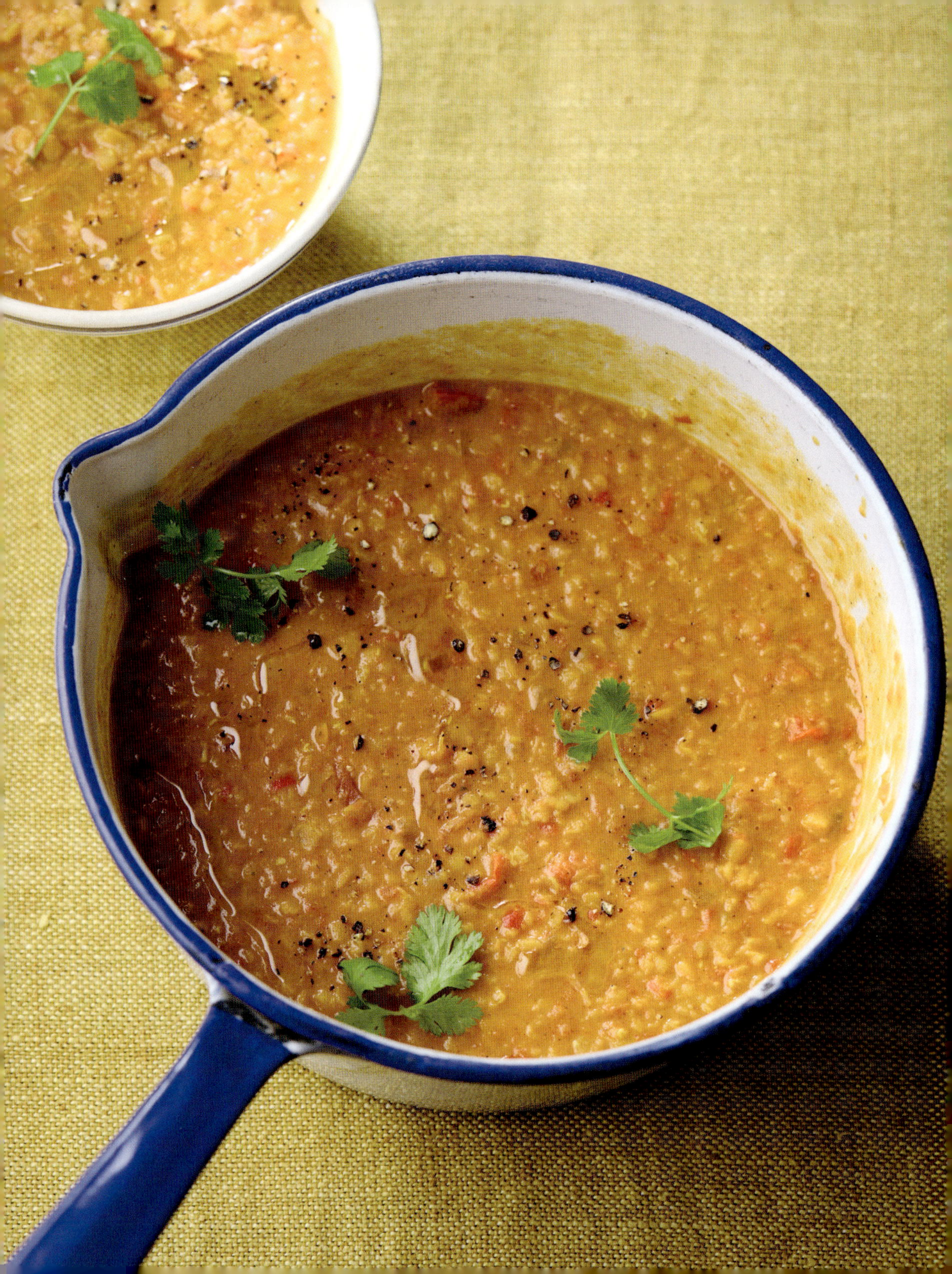

Curried Lentil Soup

Protein per serving: 17g **Kcals per serving: 463**

Serves 4

Prep + cook time: 30 minutes

- 1 tbsp extra virgin olive oil
- 1 red onion, finely chopped
- 3 cloves of garlic, crushed
- 2cm (¾in) piece of ginger, finely chopped
- 1 tbsp curry powder
- 3 large tomatoes, roughly chopped
- 400g (14oz) can of chopped tomatoes
- 400ml (14oz) can of coconut milk
- 500ml (2 cups) vegetable stock
- 200g (generous 1 cup) red lentils
- large handful of coriander, roughly chopped, plus a few leaves to serve
- juice of 1 lime
- salt

1 Add the olive oil to a large saucepan, then set over a medium-high heat. Once hot, add the onion and cook for 5 minutes until softened.

2 Add the garlic, ginger, curry powder, and fresh tomatoes, then cook for a further 3 minutes until fragrant.

3 Add the chopped tomatoes, coconut milk, and stock. Bring to the boil, add the red lentils, and reduce the heat to low. Cook for 20 minutes until the lentils are tender.

4 Add the coriander, lime juice, and a large pinch of salt, then mix well and serve with extra coriander leaves.

Swap it: Split peas also work very well here. Just be sure to add a few more minutes to the cooking time.

This tomato-rich soup is packed with plant protein, fibre, and lycopene – supporting heart health, gut function, and immune resilience in one comforting, nourishing bowl.

Seeded Cottage Cheese Bread

Protein per serving: 16g **Kcals per serving: 312**

Serves 6

Prep + cook time: 1 hour and 10 minutes

- 200g (generous 2 cups) rolled oats
- 20g (2½ tbsp) flaxseeds
- 70g (½ cup) pumpkin or sunflower seeds
- 1 tbsp fennel seeds
- 1 tsp baking powder
- 300g (1⅓ cups) cottage cheese
- 3 eggs

This hearty loaf delivers protein from cottage cheese and eggs, plus fibre and healthy fats from oats and seeds.

1 Preheat the oven to 200°C (180°C fan/ 400°F/Gas 6). Line a baking tray with baking parchment.

2 Add the oats to a blender, then pulse a few times. Transfer to a bowl.

3 Add the remaining ingredients to the bowl, then mix well until combined.

4 Transfer the mix to the lined baking tray and form into a loaf shape.

5 Bake for 1 hour until cooked through and a skewer comes out clean when inserted.

6 Let cool before slicing.

Keep it: Cut into slices, freeze, and toast from frozen.

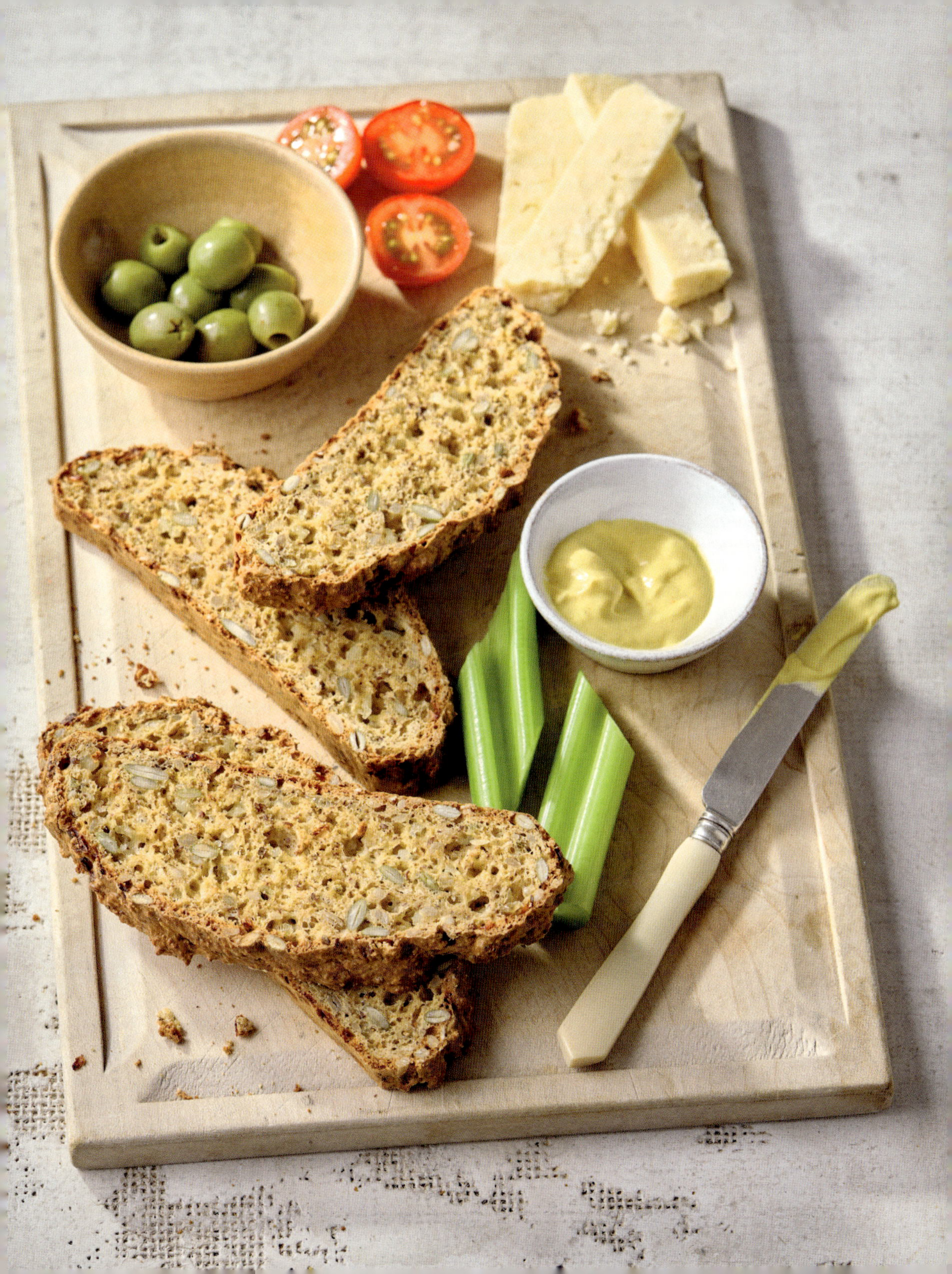

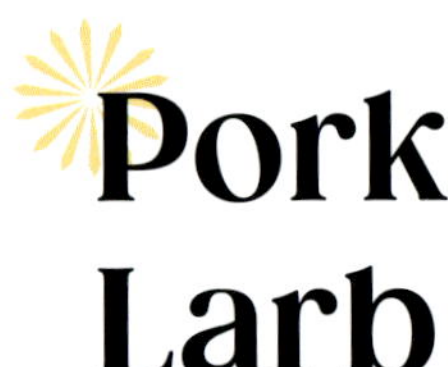

Pork Larb

Protein per serving: 26g **Kcals per serving: 287**

Serves 4

Prep + cook time: 15 minutes

Dressing:
- 1 shallot, thinly sliced
- juice of 2 limes
- 1 tbsp fish sauce
- 1 tsp maple syrup
- 2 tbsp salted peanuts, roughly chopped
- pinch of chilli flakes

Filling:
- 1 tbsp vegetable oil
- 500g (2lb 2oz) pork mince
- 1 red chilli, deseeded and finely chopped
- 1 shallot, finely chopped
- 2 spring onions, finely chopped
- 2 tbsp soy sauce

To serve:
- 3 Little Gem lettuces, leaves separated
- 2 sprigs of mint, leaves picked

1 To a small bowl, add all of the dressing ingredients, then mix well and set aside.

2 Add the oil to a large frying pan, then set over a high heat. Once hot, add the pork and cook for about 5 minutes until golden in colour.

3 Add the chilli, shallot, and spring onions to the frying pan, and cook for a further 5 minutes until softened. Add the soy sauce, mix well, turn the heat off, and set aside.

4 To serve, add the pork filling into the lettuce cups, spoon over the dressing, and sprinkle over the mint leaves.

Keep it: To batch cook for lunches, keep the dressing, filling, and lettuce separate until ready to assemble.

Swap it: Tofu works well here.

Fresh, zesty, and packed with protein, this quick pork larb delivers iron, plenty of flavour, and a satisfying crunch.

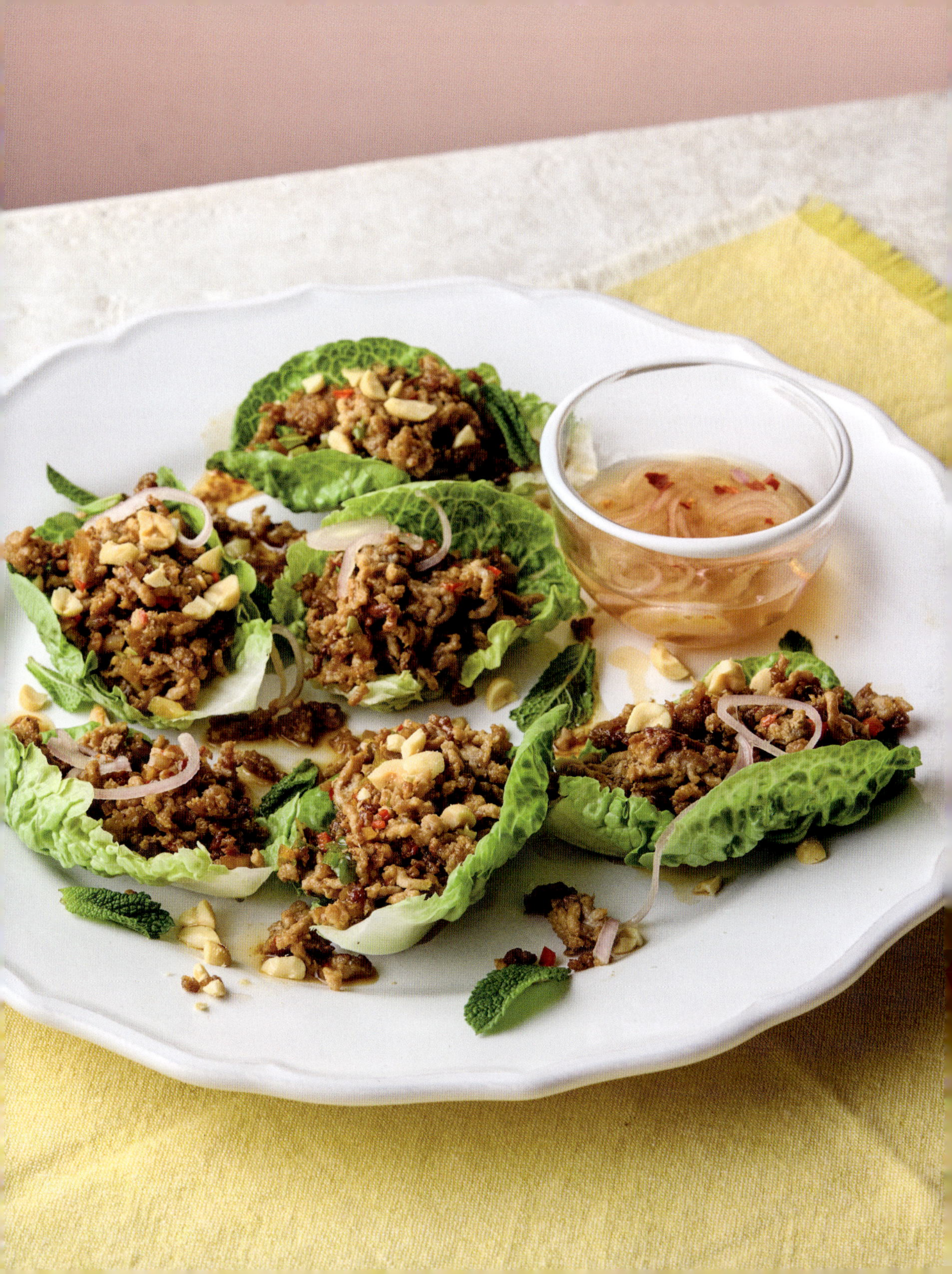

Cottage Pie

Protein per serving: 46g **Kcals per serving: 419**

Serves 4

Prep + cook time: 1 hour

- 600g (1lb 5oz) floury potatoes, peeled and cut in 3cm (1¼in) chunks
- 90ml (6 tbsp) milk
- 60g (¼ stick) unsalted butter
- 1 tbsp extra virgin olive oil
- 1 large carrot, peeled and finely chopped
- 1 stick of celery, finely chopped
- 500g (1lb 2oz) beef mince
- 1 tbsp tomato purée
- 2 tbsp gravy granules
- 1 tbsp marmite
- a few sprigs of thyme
- salt and freshly ground black pepper

1 Preheat the oven to 200°C (180°C fan/400°F/Gas 6).

2 Fill a large saucepan with cold water, then season well with salt and add the potatoes. Bring to a boil and cook for 15–20 minutes until softened. Drain, then add the potatoes back into the saucepan, along with the milk and butter. Mash with a potato masher, then set aside.

3 Meanwhile, set a saucepan over a medium heat. Add the olive oil, carrot, and celery, and cook for 10 minutes until softened.

4 Add the beef mince and cook for a further 10 minutes until golden in colour. Add the tomato purée, gravy granules, marmite, thyme, and 100ml (6½ tbsp) water. Season with salt and freshly ground black pepper, mix well, then cook for 5 minutes until the sauce is thick.

5 Transfer the beef mince to a baking dish, then top with the mashed potatoes, smoothing it over with a spoon. Cook for 25–30 minutes until golden and bubbling.

6 Top with extra black pepper and serve.

Tip: If you wish, you can save time by using ready-made mash for the topping.

This comforting classic delivers iron and protein from beef, fibre-rich veg, and a flavour boost from Marmite.

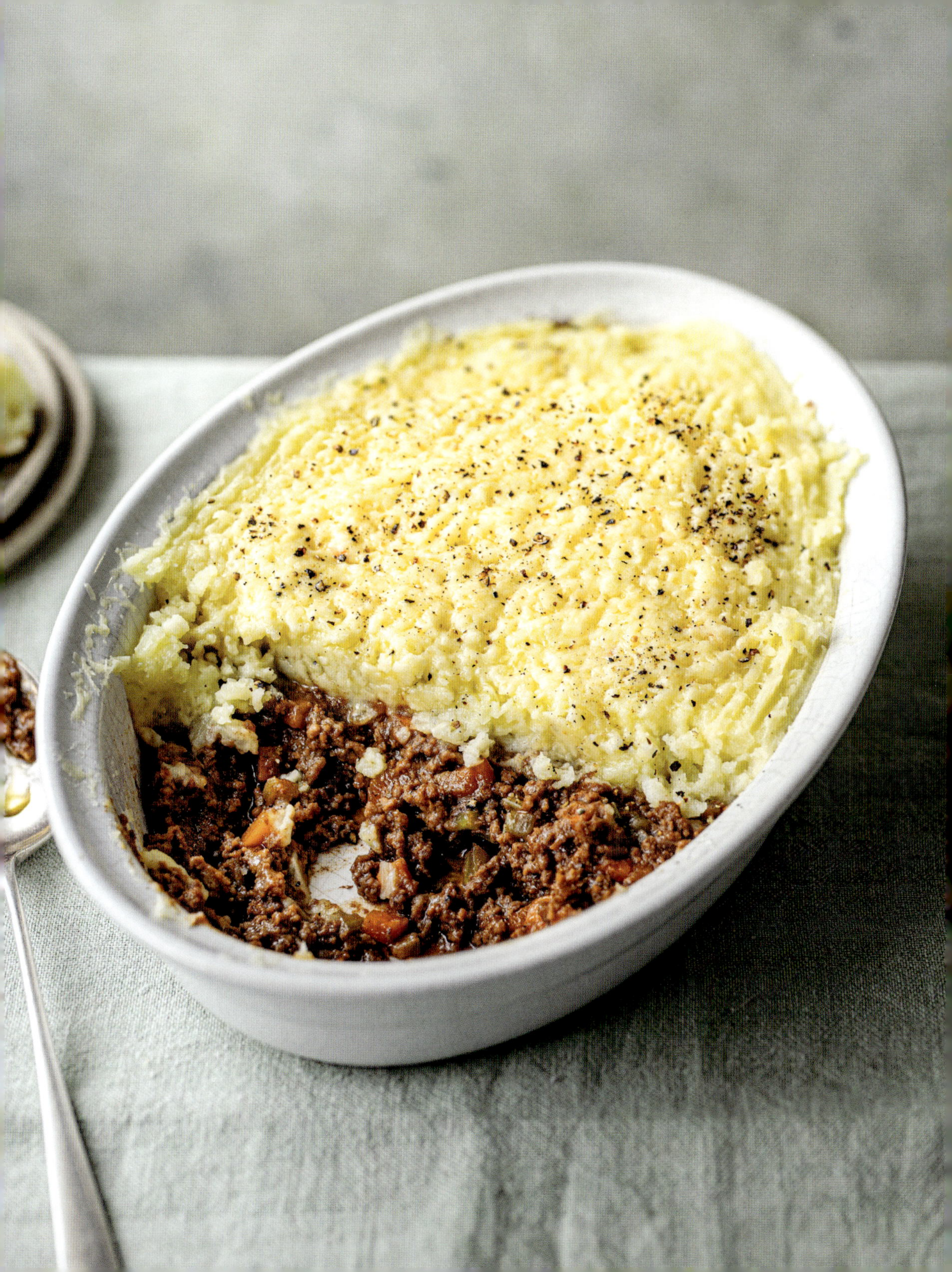

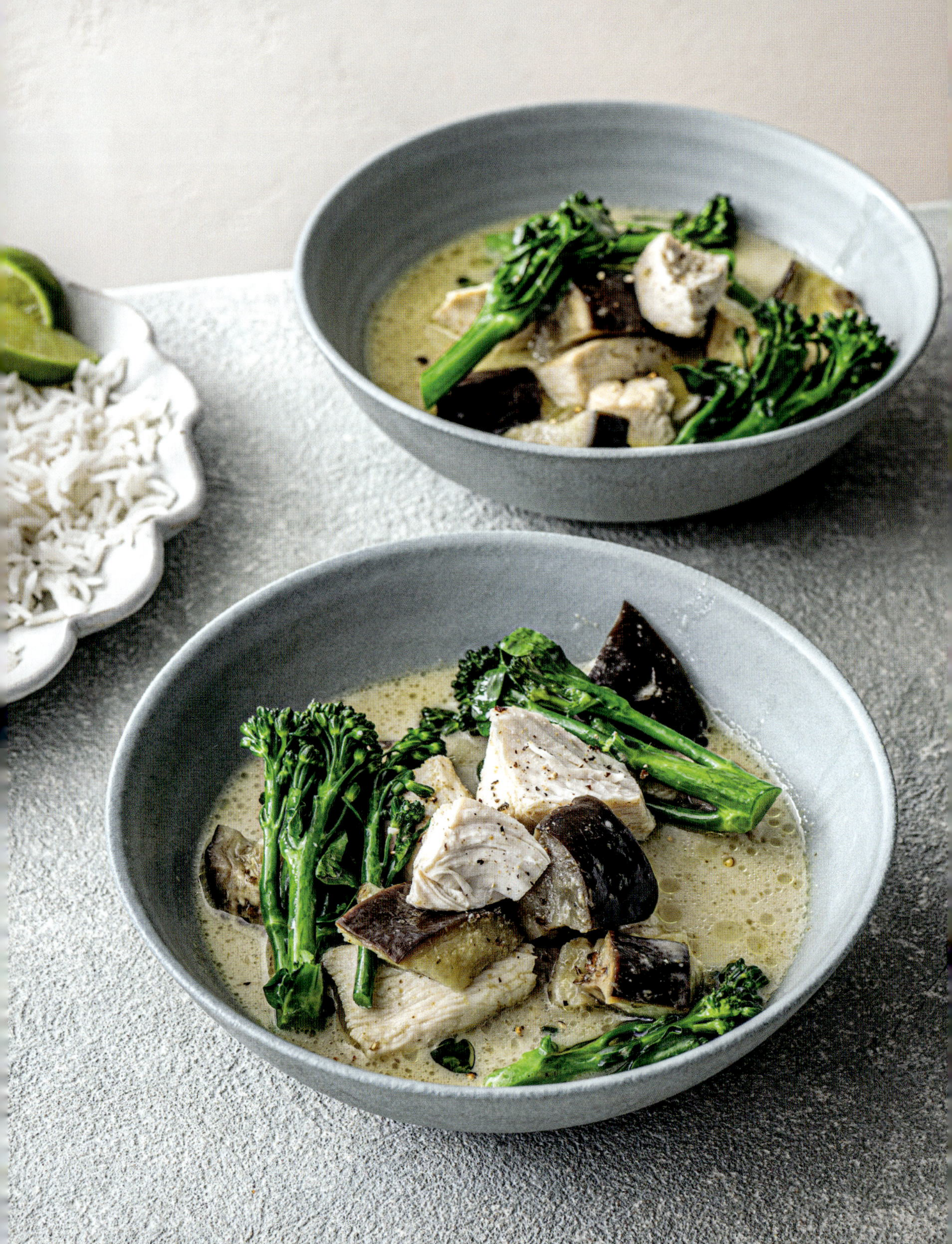

Slow Cooker Thai Green Curry

Protein per serving: 31g **Kcals per serving: 564**

Serves 4

Prep + cook time: 6 hours

- 2 tbsp Thai green curry paste
- 3 chicken breasts, cut into 4cm (1½in) chunks
- 1 aubergine, cut into 3cm (1¼in) chunks
- 400ml (14oz) can of coconut milk
- 200ml (scant 1 cup) vegetable stock
- 1 lemongrass stalk, bashed
- 1 tbsp soy sauce
- 1 tbsp fish sauce
- 1 tbsp white sugar
- 100g (3½oz) Tenderstem broccoli, halved horizontally
- juice of 2 limes

To serve (optional):

- 250g (9oz) pouch of microwaveable basmati rice
- lime wedges

1 Add all of the ingredients apart from the broccoli and lime juice into the slow cooker. Cook for 6 hours on the lowest setting. About 30 minutes before the end of the cooking time, add the broccoli.

2 Stir through the lime juice, then serve with rice and lime wedges, if liked.

Swap it: To make this vegetarian, replace the chicken with some extra veggies such as courgette or green beans, and omit the fish sauce.

Tender, lean chicken is a quality protein source, and here it is paired with fibre-rich aubergine and broccoli, supporting energy, muscle repair, and gut health.

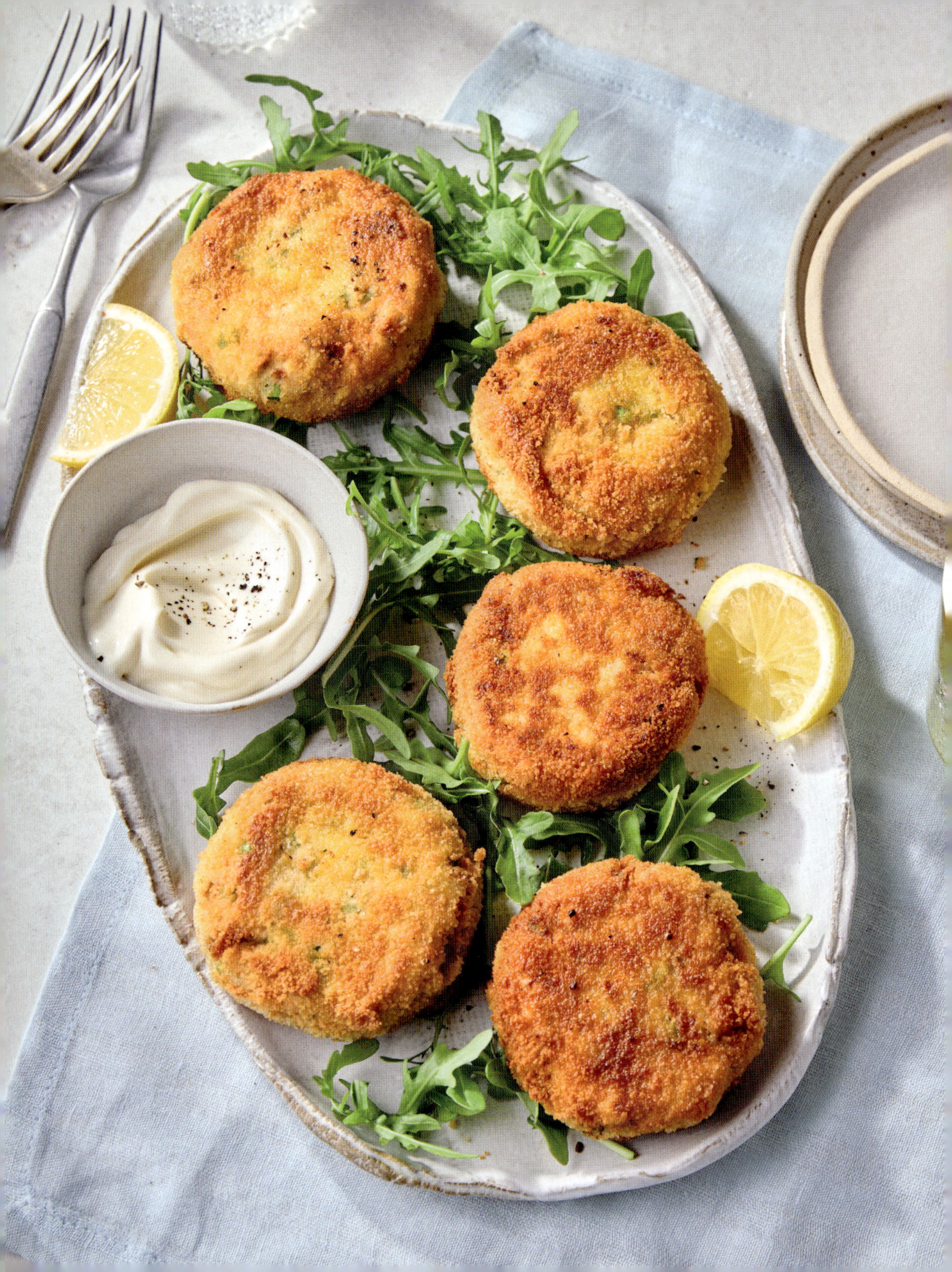

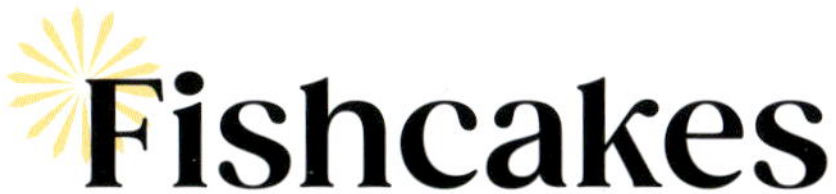

Fishcakes

Protein per serving: 35g **Kcals per serving: 449**

Serves 4

Prep + cook time: 40 minutes

- 500g (1lb 2oz) floury potatoes, peeled and cut into large chunks
- 400g (14oz) canned tuna or salmon (drained weight)
- 100g (¾ cup) frozen peas, defrosted
- handful of parsley, finely chopped
- 3 tbsp plain flour
- 2 large eggs, beaten
- 120g (1½ cups) dried breadcrumbs
- 2 tbsp vegetable oil
- salt and freshly ground black pepper

To serve (optional):

- rocket
- lemon wedges
- mayonnaise

These crispy fishcakes combine protein-rich tuna or salmon with fibre from peas and potatoes, and make a family-friendly dish.

1 Bring a large pan of salted water to the boil, add the potatoes, and cook for 10–15 minutes until softened. Drain, then pass through a ricer or mash with a fork. Set aside to cool for 10 minutes.

2 Add the tuna or salmon into the bowl with the potatoes, followed by the peas and parsley. Season with salt and freshly ground black pepper, then mix well and shape into 8 fishcakes. Set aside on a baking tray.

3 Add the flour, beaten eggs, and breadcrumbs to three separate shallow dishes.

4 Coat each fishcake in the flour, then the eggs, then the breadcrumbs.

5 Add the oil to a large frying pan set over a medium-high heat. Once hot, add the fishcakes and cook for about 3 minutes on each side until golden brown. You may need to do this in batches.

6 Remove from the pan and serve with rocket, lemon wedges, and mayonnaise, if you like.

Keep it: Keep refrigerated for 2–3 days, or freeze for up to 3 months.

Cashew Pesto Pasta

Protein per serving: 30g **Kcals per serving: 761**

Serves 4

Prep + cook time: 15 minutes

- 150g (1¼ cups) cashews
- 300g (10½oz) whole-wheat pasta
- 135g (⅔ cup) sun-dried tomato pesto
- juice of 1 lemon
- ½ clove of garlic, crushed
- 250g (9oz) pouch of microwaveable puy lentils
- 400g (14oz) can of chickpeas, drained and rinsed
- 70g (2½oz) rocket
- 3 tbsp pumpkin seeds
- salt and freshly ground black pepper

1 Put the cashews in a small bowl, cover with cold water, and set aside for 10 minutes. This is not essential, but, if you have time, it will create a creamier sauce.

2 Fill a saucepan with water, salt well, and bring to the boil. Once boiling, add the pasta and cook according to the packet instructions.

3 Meanwhile, to a blender add the cashews, pesto, lemon juice, garlic, and a pinch of salt and freshly ground black pepper. Blitz until smooth, then set aside.

4 Reserve a cup of pasta water, then drain the pasta and add the pasta back into the pan. Add the sauce, puy lentils, chickpeas, and rocket.

5 Mix well, divide among plates, and sprinkle over the pumpkin seeds.

Swap it: Other nuts, such as walnuts, would also work well here.

This speedy, bowl is packed with protein from lentils and chickpeas, fibre from whole-wheat pasta and rocket, and crunch from cashews.

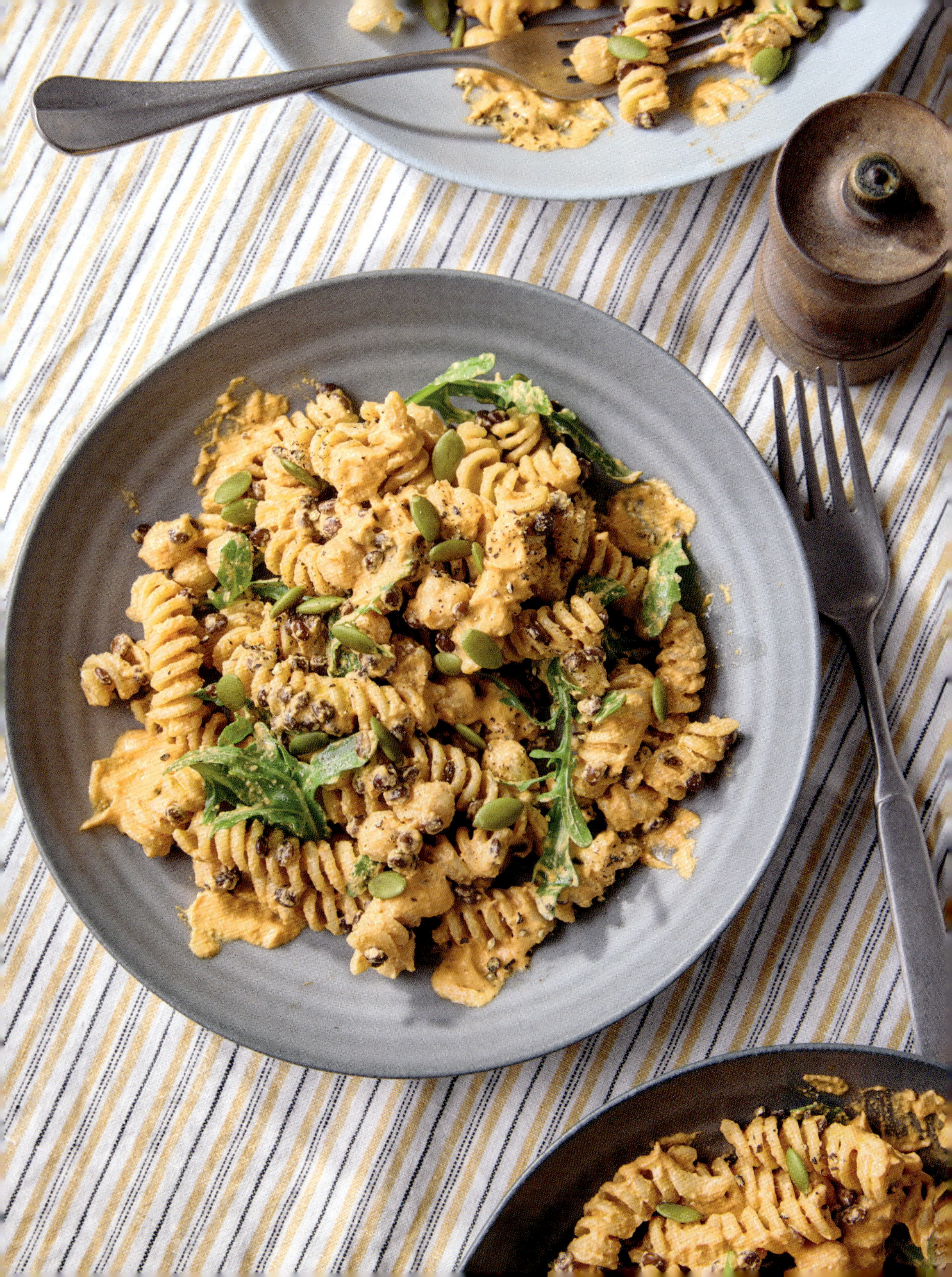

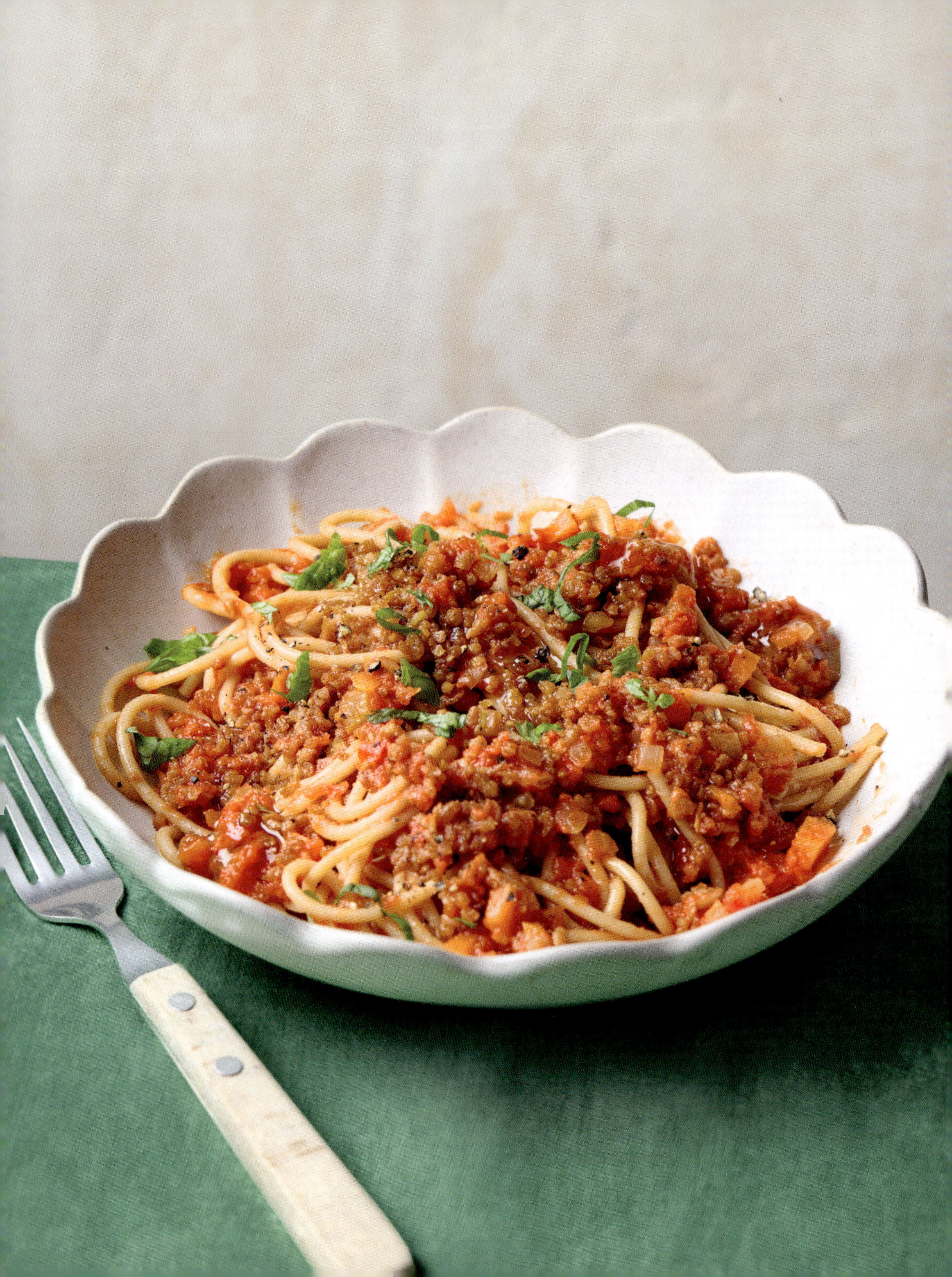

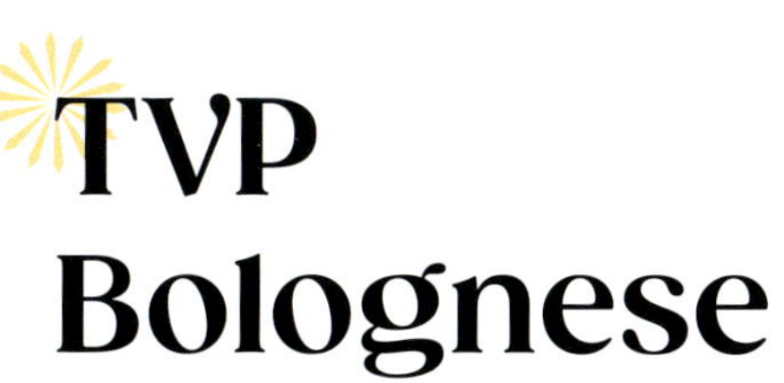

TVP Bolognese

Protein per serving: 26g **Kcals per serving: 488**

Serves 4

Prep + cook time: 40 minutes

- 2 tbsp bouillon powder
- 400ml (1¾ cups) boiling water
- 100g (3½oz) TVP (see Tip)
- 1 tbsp extra virgin olive oil
- 1 carrot, peeled and finely chopped
- 1 celery stick, finely chopped
- 1 onion, finely chopped
- 3 cloves of garlic, crushed
- 2 x 400g (14oz) cans of chopped tomatoes
- 350g (12oz) whole-wheat spaghetti
- 1 tbsp balsamic vinegar
- handful of basil, roughly chopped
- salt and freshly ground black pepper

This dish offers plant-based protein, fibre, and veg in a hearty, meat-free twist on a classic.

1 Add the bouillon powder and boiling water to a measuring jug and stir well.

2 Put the TVP in a bowl and pour the boiling stock over it. Let it sit for 3 minutes.

3 Meanwhile, to a high-sided frying pan, add the olive oil and set over a medium heat. Add the carrot, celery, onion, and garlic. Cook for about 10 minutes until softened.

4 Drain the TVP into a sieve and squeeze the liquid out with the back of a spoon. Add the TVP to the pan and cook for 5 minutes until golden in colour.

5 Add the chopped tomatoes to the pan and bring to the boil. Lower the heat to a gentle simmer and cook for about 15 minutes until the liquid has reduced.

6 Meanwhile, fill a large saucepan with water and bring to the boil. Once boiling, add the pasta and cook according to the packet instructions.

7 Once the sauce has reduced, add the balsamic vinegar and most of the basil. Season well with salt and pepper.

8 Drain the pasta, stir through the sauce, and serve topped with the remaining basil.

Tip: TVP is a soy protein that is a great substitute for meat. If non-veggie, you can use beef mince.

Slow Cooker Beef Bone Broth

Protein per 250ml (1 cup): 7g

Kcals per 250ml (1 cup): 100

Makes 2.5 litres (10 cups)

Prep + cook time: 12 hours 45 minutes

- 2kg (4½lb) beef bones
- 1 onion, cut into chunks
- 2 carrots, roughly chopped
- 2 celery sticks, roughly chopped
- 2 tbsp apple cider vinegar
- 1 bulb of garlic, halved
- 5 peppercorns
- 2 star anise
- salt and freshly ground black pepper

1 Preheat the oven to 200°C (180°C fan/ 400°F/Gas 6).

2 Put the beef bones on a baking tray and roast for 40 minutes until they are a dark brown colour.

3 Add the roasted bones to a slow cooker, then top with the remaining ingredients.

4 Fill the slow cooker with cold water so that it covers the ingredients. Set the slow cooker on low, and leave to cook for 12 hours.

5 Strain, then it's ready to use.

Keep it: Refrigerate for up to 5 days. Freeze for up to 3 months.

This slow-cooked beef bone broth is rich in collagen, gelatine, and minerals that support joint, gut, and skin health.

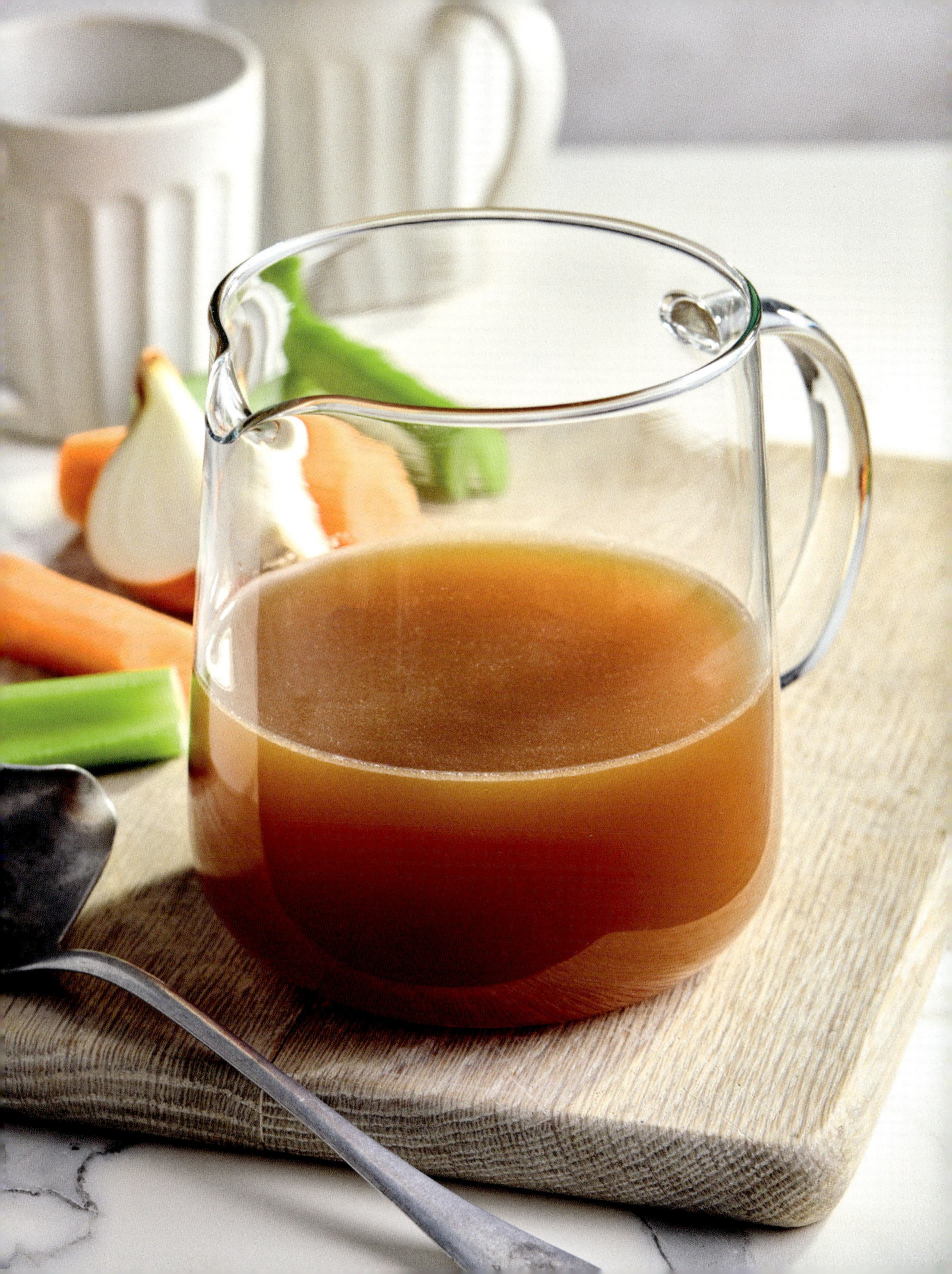

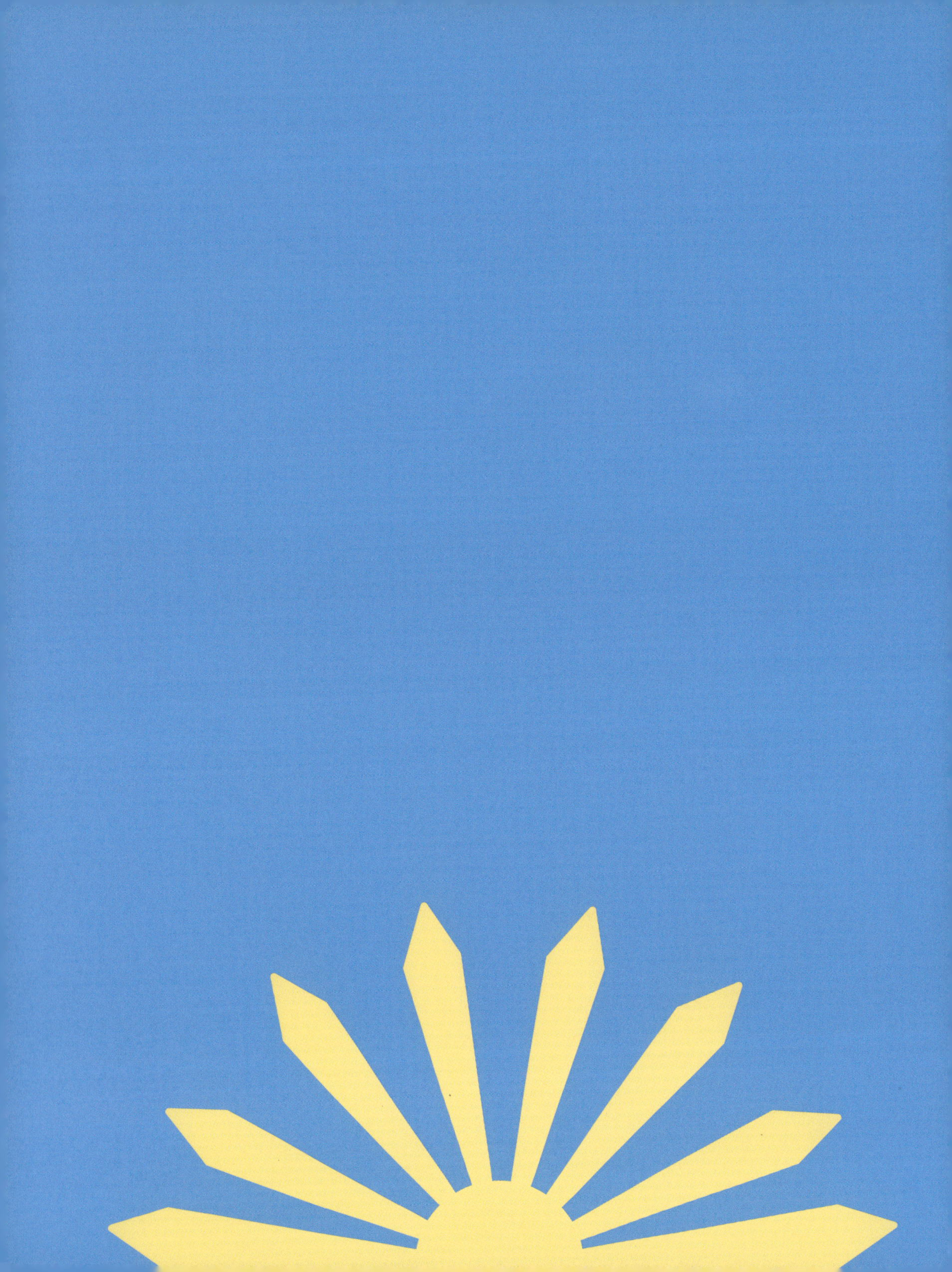

Air Fryer

Even if you haven't had time to do any meal prep, with the help of an air fryer, you can whip up a protein-packed meal in no time. These are also recipes that are perfect when you want to give yourself a treat – by using a fraction of the oil, you can enjoy things like crispy buffalo wings or prawn toast guilt free!

Chicken Caesar Salad

Protein per serving: 32g **Kcals per serving: 480**

Serves 4

Prep + cook time: 35 minutes

- 50g (1¾oz) seeded sourdough bread, cut into 2cm (¾in) pieces
- 4 large eggs
- 4 streaky bacon rashers
- 4 skin-on chicken thighs
- 2 large tomatoes, roughly chopped
- 2 Little Gem lettuces, or 1 large romaine lettuce, cut into large chunks
- vegetable or olive oil cooking spray
- salt and freshly ground black pepper

Dressing:

- 100g (scant ½ cup) Greek yogurt
- 2 tbsp mayonnaise
- 2 tsp Dijon mustard
- juice of ½ lemon
- 3 anchovy fillets
- 20g (scant ⅓ cup) finely grated Parmesan
- 1 clove of garlic, crushed

1 Preheat the air fryer to 180°C/350°F for 3 minutes.

2 Add the bread and eggs (in their shells) to the air fryer basket and spray the bread with oil. Cook at 180°C/350°F for 8 minutes. Set both aside.

3 Add the bacon to the air fryer basket. Cook at 180°C/350°F for 7 minutes. Set aside.

4 Add the chicken to the air fryer basket, skin-side up, and cook at 180°C/350°F for 15 minutes until golden in colour and cooked through. Set aside.

5 Meanwhile, add all of the dressing ingredients to a blender and blitz until smooth. Set aside.

6 Roughly chop the bacon, then add to a bowl. Slice the chicken into small pieces, then add to the bowl. Add in the tomatoes, lettuce, sourdough croutons, and the dressing, then mix well. Peel and halve the eggs, then arrange on top. Sprinkle over a little salt and pepper to serve.

Tip: You can be flexible with this salad if you don't have all the ingredients.

Along with the chicken, bacon, and eggs, the cleverly designed dressing gives this dish an extra protein boost.

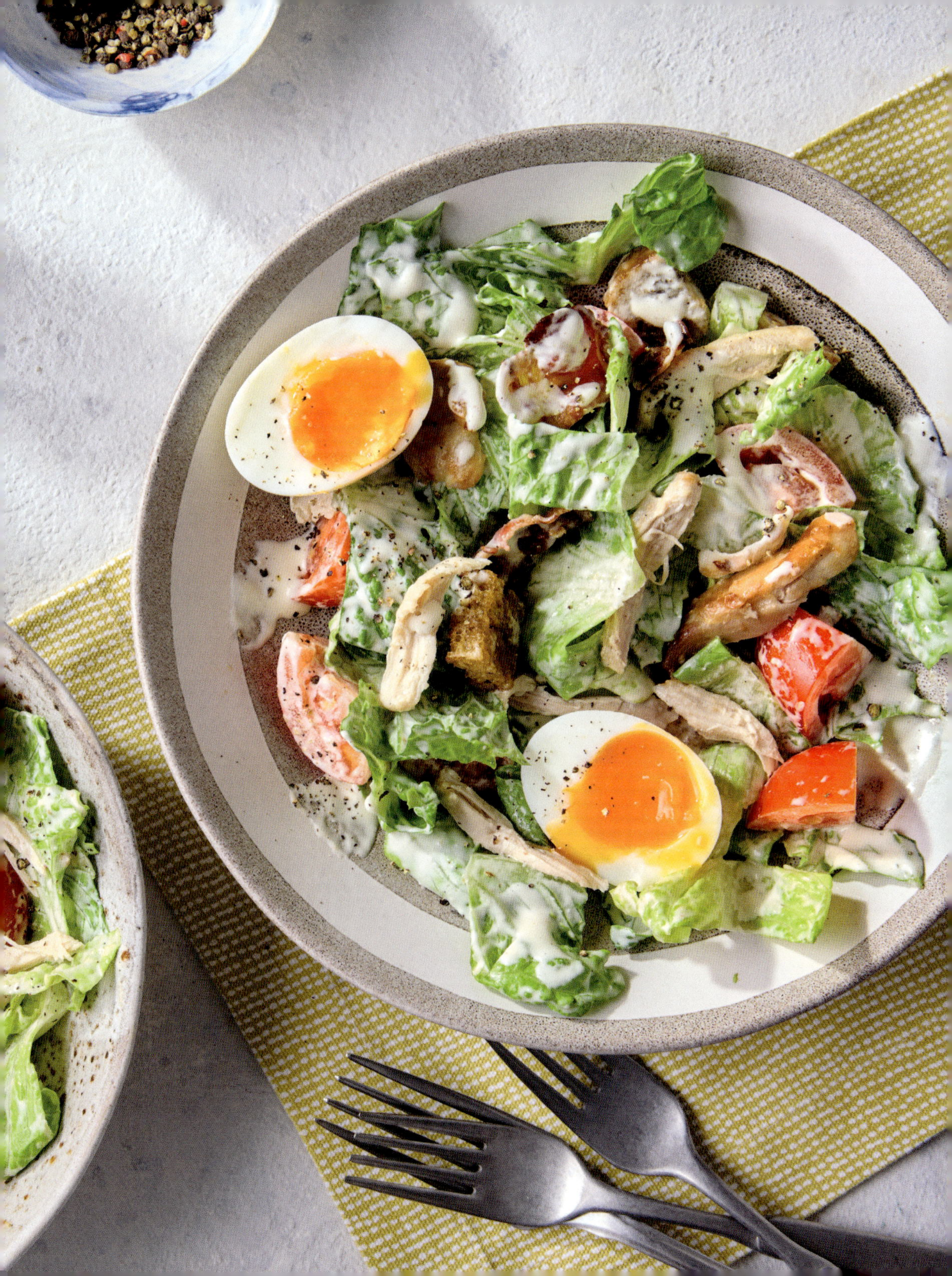

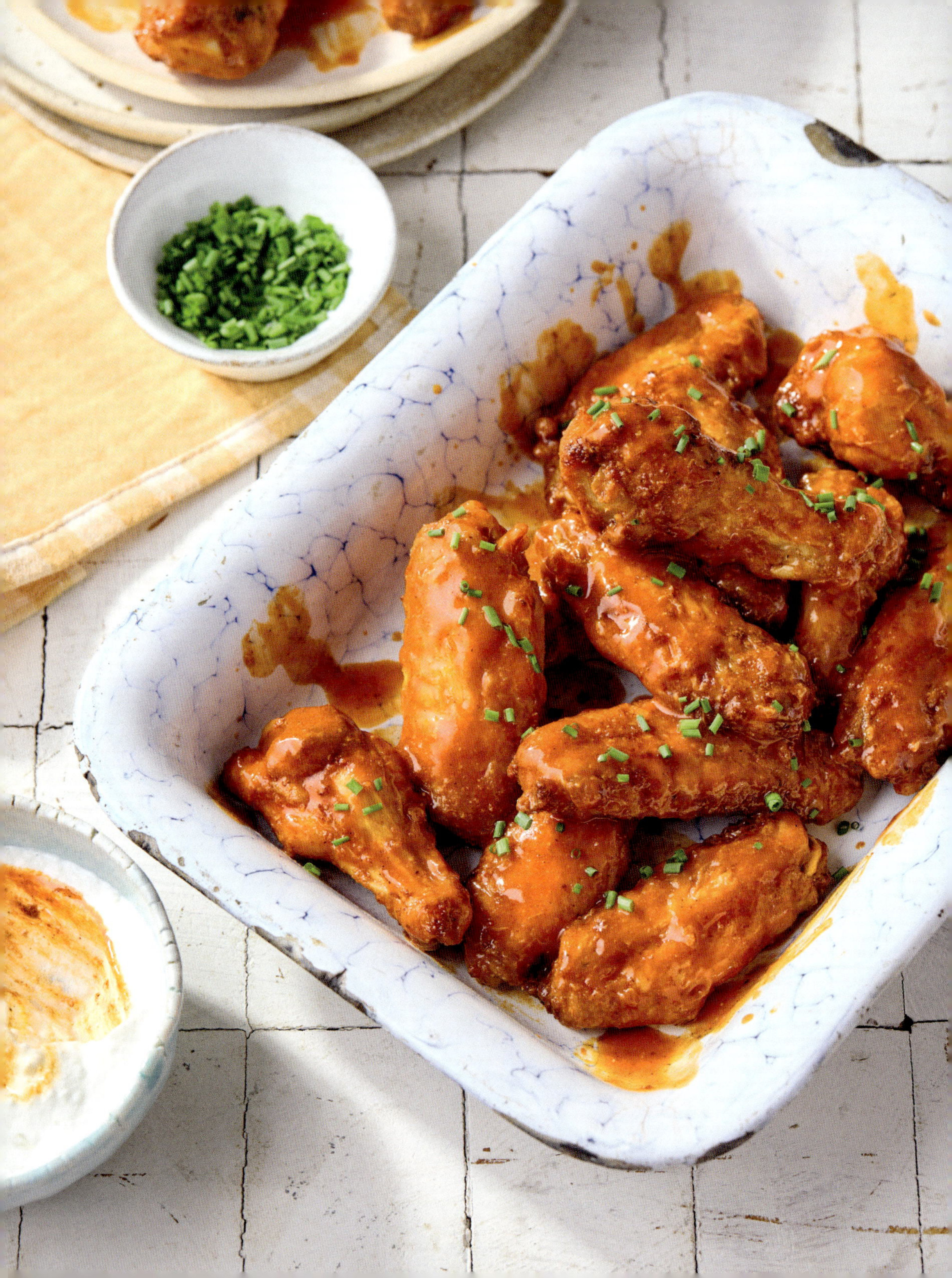

Buffalo Chicken Wings

Protein per serving: 39g **Kcals per serving: 450**

Serves 4

Prep + cook time: 30 minutes

- 1kg (2¼lb) chicken wings, wing tips trimmed and halved through the joint
- 1 tsp smoked paprika
- 2 tsp baking powder
- 2 tsp garlic powder
- 2 tsp onion granules
- 150g (5oz) buffalo hot sauce
- 20g (1½ tbsp) butter
- 200g (scant 1 cup) cottage cheese
- handful of chives, finely chopped
- vegetable or olive oil cooking spray

These spicy wings are packed with protein, while the cottage cheese dip adds calcium and a lighter twist on the classic pairing.

1 Preheat the air fryer to 190°C/375°F for 3 minutes.

2 Add the chicken wings to a bowl and dry them well with some kitchen paper.

3 Add the paprika, baking powder, 1 teaspoon garlic powder, and 1 teaspoon onion granules. Mix well.

4 Working in batches, if necessary, arrange the wings in the air fryer basket, skin-side up, in a single layer. Spray liberally with oil, then cook at 190°C/375°F for 15 minutes until crispy.

5 Meanwhile, to a small saucepan, add the hot sauce and butter. Cook over a low-medium heat until the butter has melted and the sauce starts to bubble. Transfer to a bowl and set aside.

6 To a blender, add the cottage cheese, the remaining 1 teaspoon garlic powder, and 1 teaspoon onion granules, then blitz until smooth. Set aside.

7 Toss the chicken wings through the buffalo sauce, then sprinkle over the chives and serve with the cottage cheese dip.

Swap it: Feel free to swap the buffalo sauce for your preferred wing sauce. Soy and honey would also be a great combo.

Crispy Aubergines with Chickpea Salad

Protein per serving: 38g **Kcals per serving: 797**

Serves 2

Prep + cook time: 40 minutes

- 2 aubergines
- 400g (14oz) can of chickpeas, drained and rinsed
- ½ cucumber, roughly chopped
- 200g (7oz) pomegranate seeds
- ½ red onion, finely chopped
- 1 large tomato, roughly chopped
- 1 tsp dried oregano
- 1 tbsp extra virgin olive oil
- juice of 1 lemon
- 2 tbsp plain flour
- 1 large egg, beaten
- 100g (2⅓ cups) panko breadcrumbs
- 100g (3½oz) feta
- 2 tbsp Greek yogurt
- vegetable or olive oil cooking spray
- salt and freshly ground black pepper

1 Preheat the air fryer to 220°C/425°F for 3 minutes.

2 Put the whole aubergines in the air fryer basket and cook at 220°C/425°F for 10 minutes until softened. Transfer to a bowl, cover with cling film, and let cool slightly for 5 minutes.

3 Meanwhile, combine the chickpeas, cucumber, pomegranate seeds, red onion, tomato, oregano, olive oil, and lemon juice in a bowl. Season with salt and pepper, then set aside.

4 Add the flour, beaten egg, and panko breadcrumbs to three separate shallow dishes.

5 Peel the skins off the aubergines. Coat each aubergine first in the flour, then the egg, then the breadcrumbs.

6 Put into the air fryer basket, spray well with oil, then cook at 190°C/375°F for 10 minutes. Flip them over, spray with some more oil, and cook at 190°C/375°F for a further 10 minutes until golden and crispy.

7 Meanwhile, to a blender, add the feta, Greek yogurt, and 2 tablespoons water. Season with salt and pepper, then blitz until smooth.

8 To serve, spread the yogurt mixture out onto a plate, top with the chickpea salad, then arrange the aubergines on top.

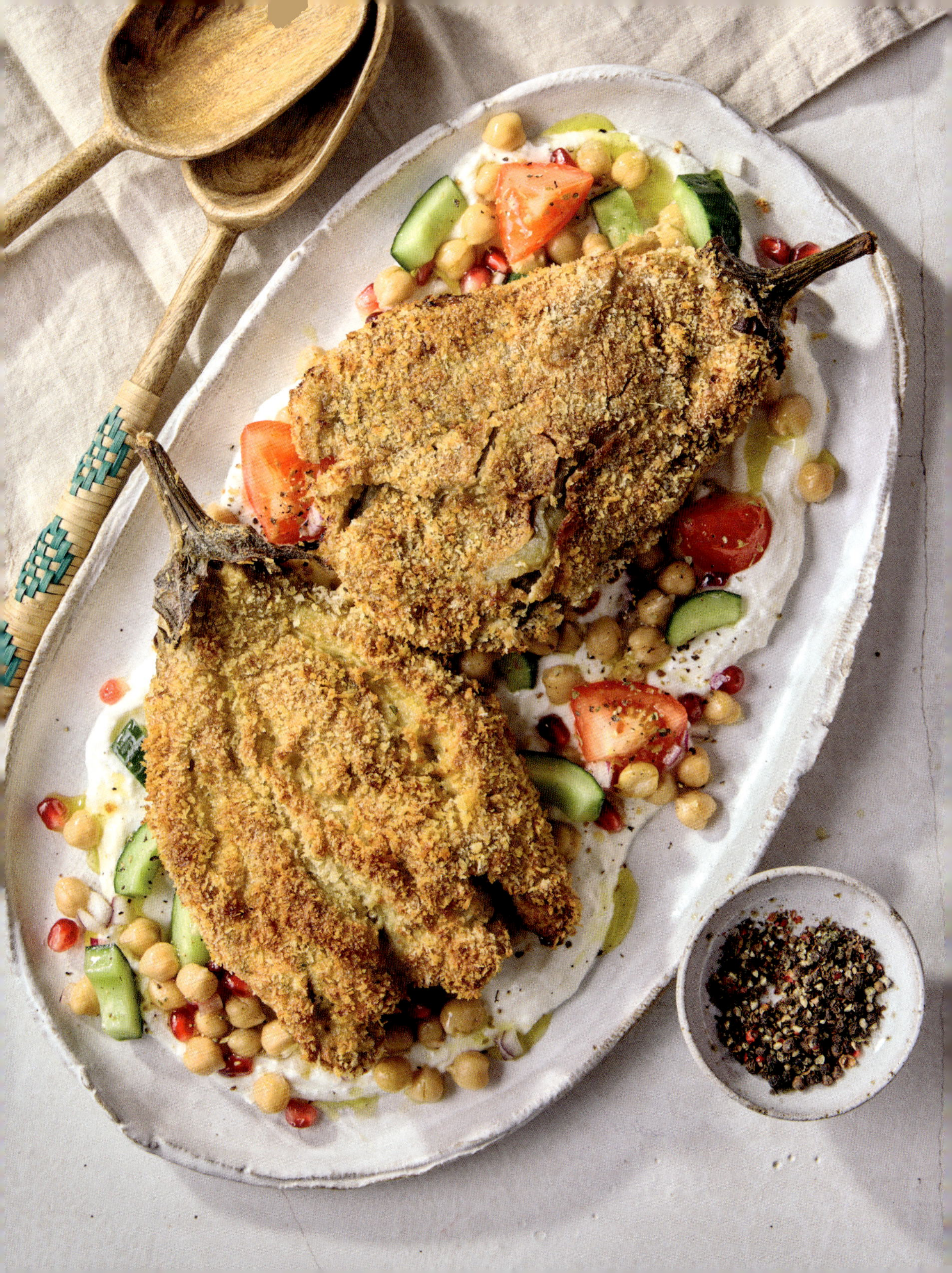

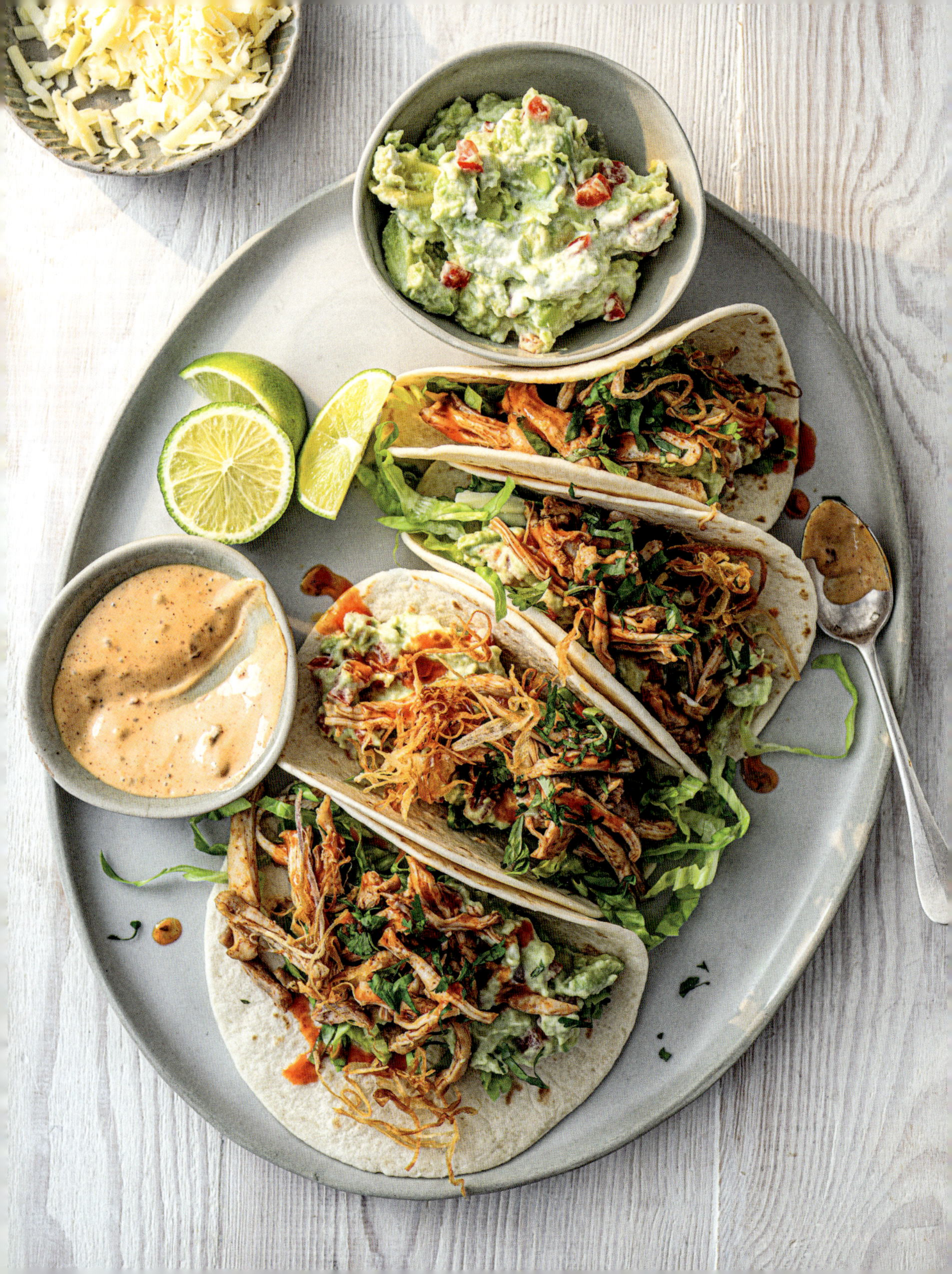

Chicken Tacos

Protein per serving: 38g **Kcals per serving: 795**

Serves 4

Prep + cook time: 15 minutes

- 4 boneless, skinless chicken thighs
- 1 tbsp fajita seasoning
- 2 tbsp extra virgin olive oil
- 2 avocados
- 1 tbsp soured cream
- juice of 1 lime
- 1 large tomato, deseeded and finely chopped
- handful of coriander, roughly chopped
- 50g (scant ¼ cup) mayonnaise
- 1 tsp chipotle paste
- 6–8 small tortilla wraps
- 1 Little Gem lettuce, shredded
- 50g (½ cup) grated Cheddar
- small handful of crispy friend onions
- salt and freshly ground black pepper

These tacos bring together juicy chicken, creamy avocado, and crunchy lettuce for a nice mix of protein, healthy fats, and fresh veg.

1 Preheat the air fryer to 180°C/350°F for 3 minutes.

2 To a bowl, add the chicken thighs, fajita seasoning, and olive oil. Season with salt and freshly ground black pepper, then mix well.

3 Add the chicken to the air fryer basket, then cook at 180°C/350°F for 10 minutes until the chicken is nicely charred and cooked through. Shred the chicken, then set aside.

4 Meanwhile, to a small bowl, add the avocados and mash with a fork. Add the soured cream, lime juice, and tomato. Season with salt, mix well, and set aside.

5 To a second small bowl, add the mayo and chipotle paste, mix well, and set aside.

6 Heat the wraps according to the packet instructions.

7 To assemble, add some of the avocado mix to a wrap and top with some chicken, chipotle mayo, Little Gem, and Cheddar, then serve.

Swap it: Elements of these tacos are easily adaptable; prawns instead of chicken work incredibly well here.

Crispy Gochujang Tempeh

Protein per serving: 28g **Kcals per serving: 459**

Serves 2

Prep + cook time: 20 minutes

- 2 tbsp plain flour
- 50ml (3½ tbsp) milk of choice
- 100g (2⅓ cups) panko breadcrumbs
- 200g (7oz) tempeh, torn into small pieces
- 2 tbsp gochujang
- 1 tbsp maple syrup
- 1 tbsp soy sauce
- 1 tsp rice vinegar
- 1 spring onion, thinly sliced
- 1 tbsp sesame seeds
- vegetable or olive oil cooking spray

This crispy tempeh brings bold flavour and plant-based protein, ready to be accompanied by whatever you fancy.

1 Preheat the air fryer to 200°C/400°F for 3 minutes.

2 Add the plain flour and milk to a small bowl, whisk well, and set aside. Add the panko to another small bowl and set aside.

3 Add the tempeh pieces to the wet batter to coat, then toss the pieces in the panko until fully coated.

4 Arrange in the air fryer basket, spray with some oil, and cook at 200°C/400°F for 15 minutes until crispy.

5 Meanwhile, add the gochujang, maple syrup, soy sauce, and rice vinegar to a bowl, whisk well, and set aside.

6 Add the tempeh to the gochujang glaze, toss well so the pieces are fully coated in the sauce, then sprinkle over the spring onion and sesame seeds.

Serve it: To make this more of a meal, serve with any grain you prefer, and some veggies. Cucumber, tomato, and green beans work well.

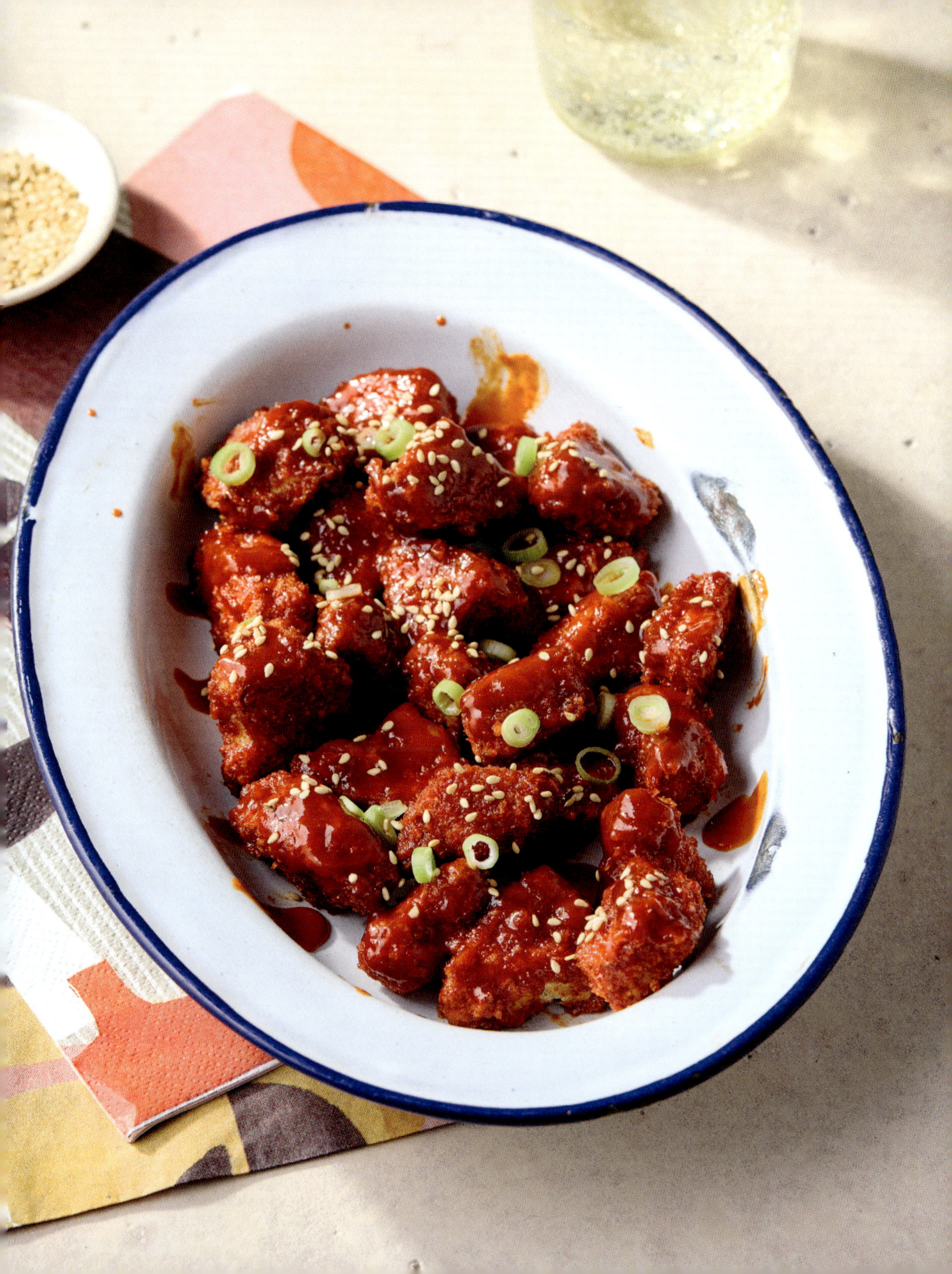

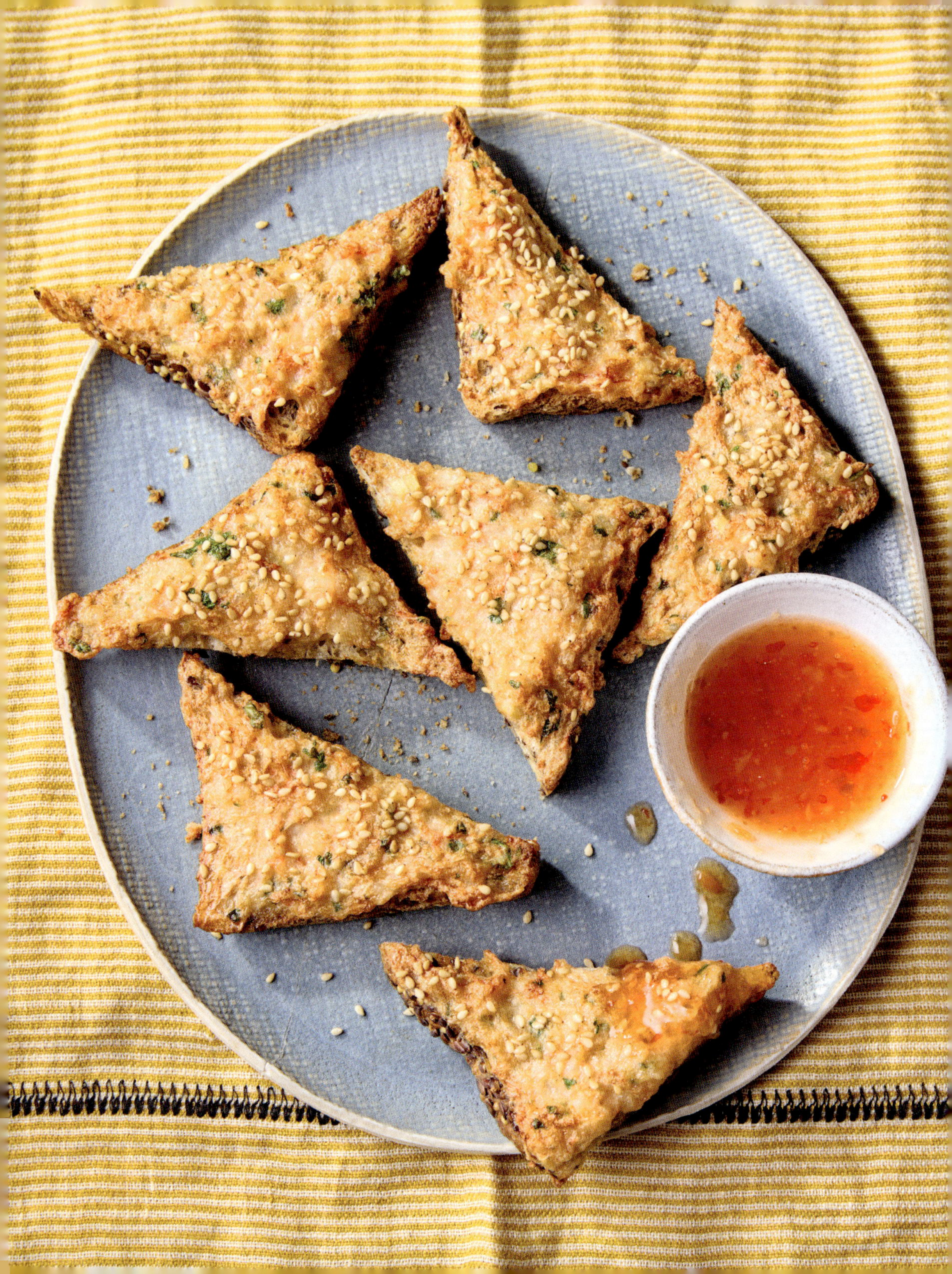

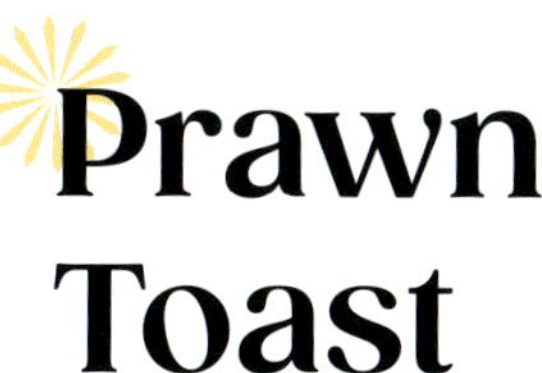

Prawn Toast

Protein per serving: 24g **Kcals per serving: 296**

Serves 2

Prep + cook time: 15 minutes

- 3 tbsp black and white sesame seeds
- 165g (6oz) raw king prawns
- 1 spring onion, finely chopped
- 1 tsp garlic powder
- 2cm (¾in) piece of ginger, finely chopped
- 1 tbsp soy sauce
- 1 egg white
- handful of coriander, roughly chopped
- 2 slices of seeded sourdough bread
- vegetable or olive oil cooking spray
- salt

To serve (optional):

sweet chilli sauce

1 Preheat the air fryer to 190°C/375°F for 3 minutes.

2 Put the sesame seeds onto a small baking tray and set aside.

3 To a blender, add the prawns, spring onion, garlic powder, ginger, soy sauce, egg white, and coriander. Season with a little salt, then blitz until smooth.

4 Spread the prawn paste over the slices of sourdough. Press the bread, prawn paste-side down, into the sesame seeds so that they stick to the prawn paste.

5 Put the slices into the air fryer basket, prawn paste-side up, then spray with some oil and cook at 190°C/375°F for 8 minutes until crispy and golden.

6 Serve with sweet chilli sauce, if liked.

Keep it: Feel free to double up this recipe and freeze any extra. They will keep in the freezer for up to 3 months.

Prawns provide lean protein, zinc, and vitamin B12, while seeded sourdough adds fibre and crunch. Quick to prep and big on flavour.

Halloumi Burgers

Protein per serving: 45g **Kcals per serving: 795**

Serves 2

Prep + cook time: 20 minutes

- 2 tbsp plain flour
- 1 egg, beaten
- 100g (2⅓ cups) panko breadcrumbs
- 2 tbsp sesame seeds
- 225g (8oz) halloumi, cut into 2 large slices
- ¼ red cabbage, finely shredded
- 1 tbsp harissa paste
- 2 tbsp Greek yogurt
- 2 burger or ciabatta buns
- vegetable or olive oil cooking spray
- salt and freshly ground black pepper

1 Preheat the air fryer to 190°C/375°F for 3 minutes.

2 Add the flour, beaten egg, and panko breadcrumbs to three separate shallow dishes. Add the sesame seeds to the panko bowl.

3 Coat each halloumi slice in the flour, then the beaten egg, and then the panko. Arrange in the air fryer basket.

4 Spray the halloumi with oil, then cook at 190°C/375°F for 10 minutes.

5 Meanwhile, put the cabbage into a bowl, season with some salt and freshly ground black pepper, and set aside.

6 To a small bowl, add the harissa and yogurt, then season with salt. Mix well and set aside.

7 Cut the buns open, then spread some of the harissa yogurt onto the base. Top with the halloumi, followed by some red cabbage. Place the bun lid on top and serve.

Swap it: Paneer would also work well here.

Halloumi provides satisfying protein with its creamy texture and bonus nutrients like calcium and phosphorus for bone health.

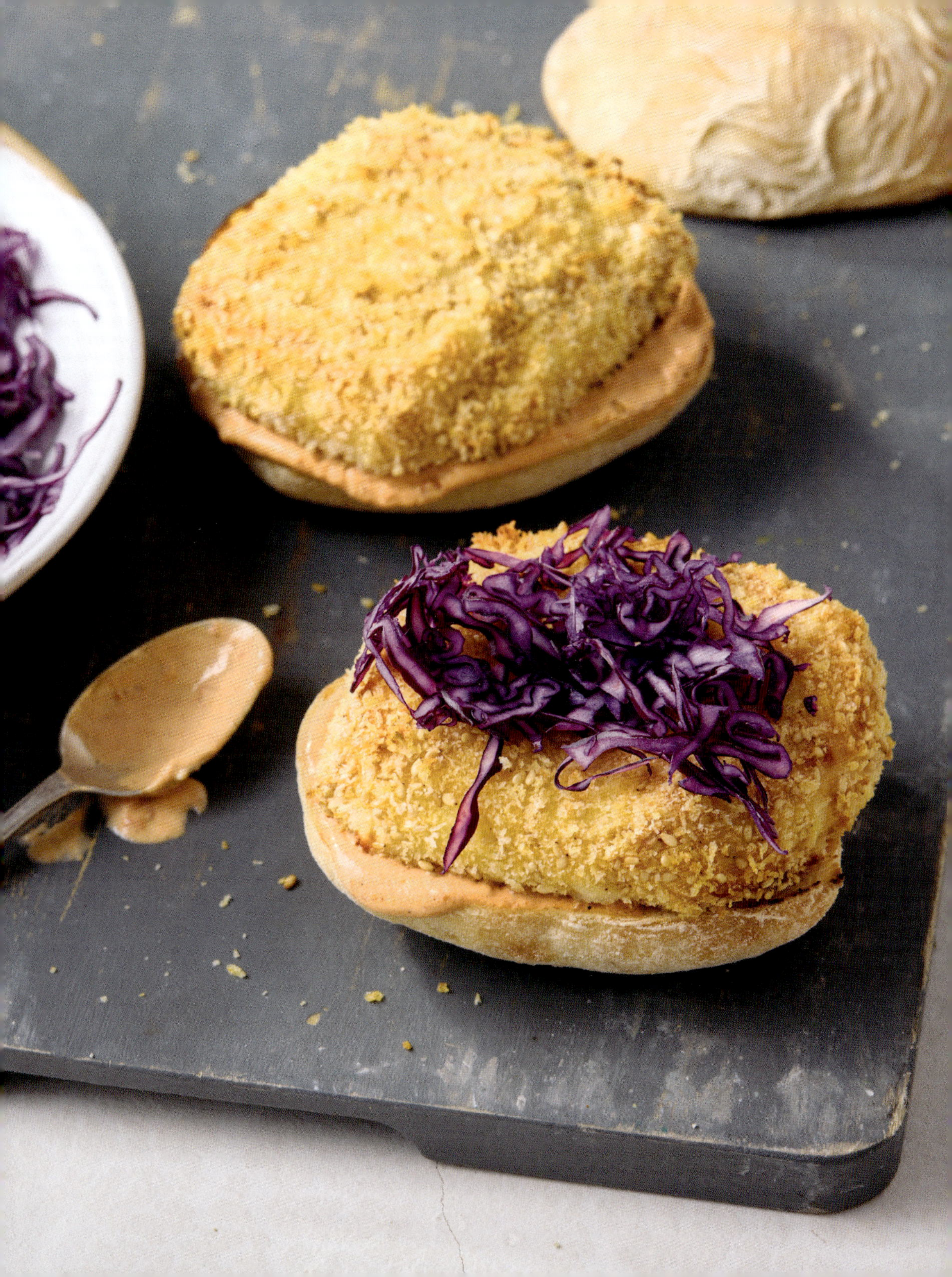

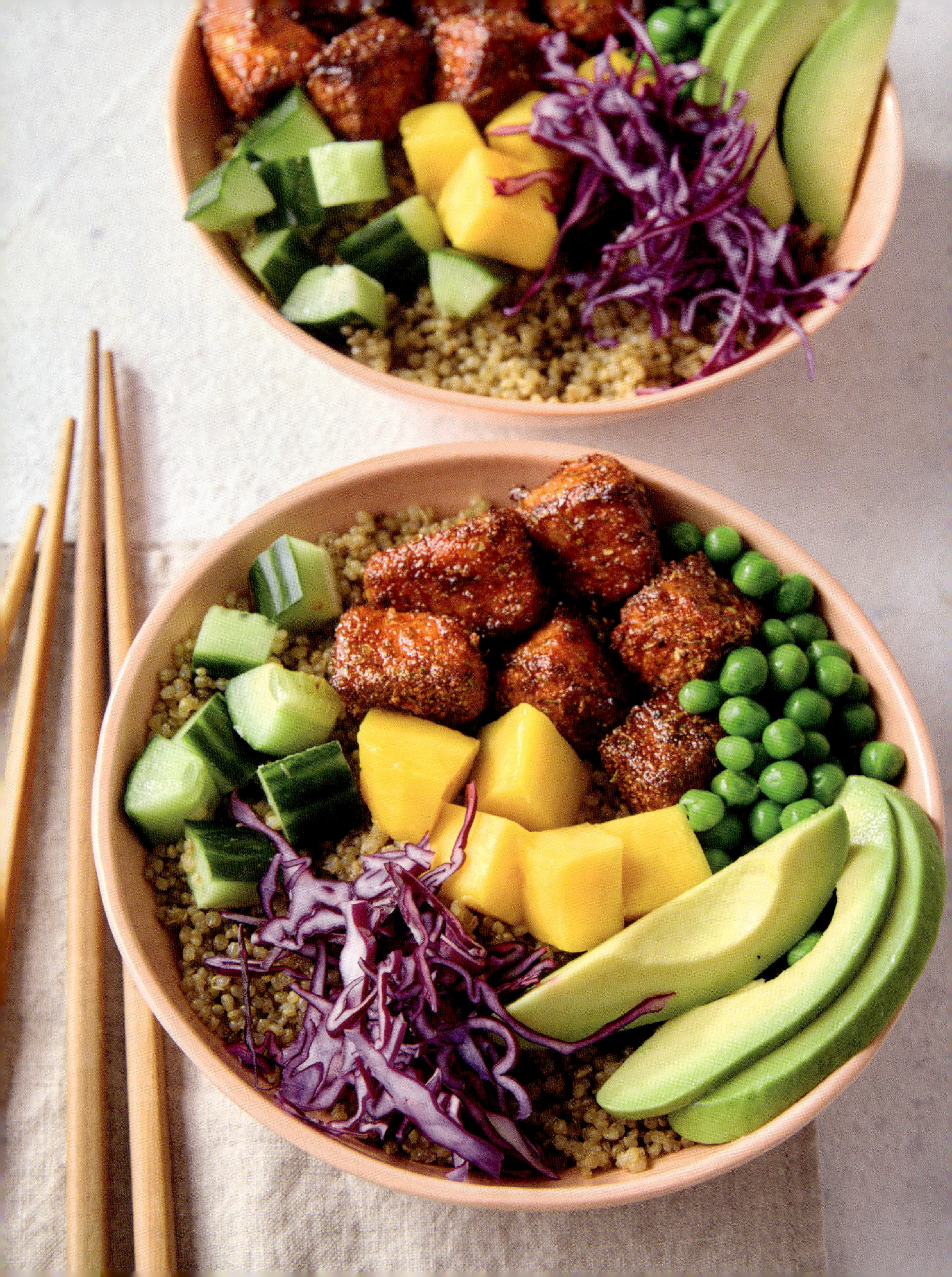

Blackened Salmon Bowl

Protein per serving: 40g **Kcals per serving: 740**

Serves 2

Prep + cook time: 15 minutes

- 2 skinless salmon fillets, cut into 4cm (1½in) pieces
- 1 tbsp paprika
- 1 tsp garlic granules
- 1 tsp onion powder
- 1 tsp dried oregano
- 1 tsp light soft brown sugar
- 250g (9oz) pouch of microwaveable quinoa
- 1 mango, peeled, stoned, and roughly chopped
- 1 avocado, roughly chopped
- 100g (¾ cup) frozen peas, defrosted
- ½ cucumber, roughly chopped
- ¼ red cabbage, finely shredded
- juice of 1 lime
- vegetable or olive oil cooking spray
- salt and freshly ground black pepper

1 Preheat the air fryer to 200°C/400°F for 3 minutes.

2 Add the salmon to a bowl, then add in the paprika, garlic granules, onion powder, oregano, and sugar. Season with salt and freshly ground black pepper. Mix well to coat the salmon.

3 Put the salmon in the air fryer basket, spray with some oil, then cook at 200°C/400°F for 5 minutes until cooked through.

4 Meanwhile, microwave the quinoa pouch according to the packet instructions, then set aside.

5 To assemble, divide the quinoa pouch between two bowls and top with the salmon, mango, avocado, peas, cucumber, and red cabbage. Squeeze over the lime juice and serve.

Swap it: This would also work well with tofu for a vegan version.

This vibrant bowl is a colourful, nourishing mix of healthy fats, fibre, and fresh flavour.

Chicken Spring Rolls

Protein per serving: 25g **Kcals per serving: 418**

Serves 4

Prep + cook time: 40 minutes

- 1 tbsp vegetable oil
- 300g (10½oz) chicken mince
- 2 cloves of garlic, crushed
- ¼ Chinese leaf cabbage, shredded
- 1 carrot, grated
- 1 tsp sesame oil
- 2 tbsp oyster sauce
- 135g (4¾oz) rice paper wrappers
- vegetable or olive oil cooking spray

Dipping sauce (optional):

- 3 tbsp smooth peanut butter
- 1 tbsp soy sauce
- juice of 1 lime
- 1 tsp maple syrup

These light, crispy spring rolls are filled with protein-rich chicken and fibre-packed veg – a fresh, flavourful option for a balanced lunch or snack.

1 Add the oil to a frying pan and set over a medium-high heat. Once hot, add the chicken mince and cook for 5 minutes until golden. Add the garlic, cabbage, and carrot, then cook for a further 2 minutes until softened. Stir through the sesame oil and oyster sauce, remove from the heat, and set aside to cool for 10–15 minutes.

2 Preheat the air fryer to 190°C/375°F for 3 minutes.

3 Fill a shallow bowl with lukewarm water, then briefly soak one of the rice papers in the water. Place the soaked rice paper on a chopping board. Spoon some of the mixture on the closest edge to you, then fold in both of the sides, and roll away from you. Repeat this with a second wrapper around the same roll, so it is double wrapped. Repeat with the rest of the filling and wrappers.

4 Put the spring rolls into the air fryer basket, spray with oil, and cook at 190°C/375°F for 12 minutes until crispy.

5 Combine all of the dipping sauce ingredients, if making, in a small bowl. Serve the spring rolls alongside the dipping sauce, if using.

Swap it: To make this veggie, swap the chicken mince for small pieces of tofu, and swap the oyster sauce for soy sauce.

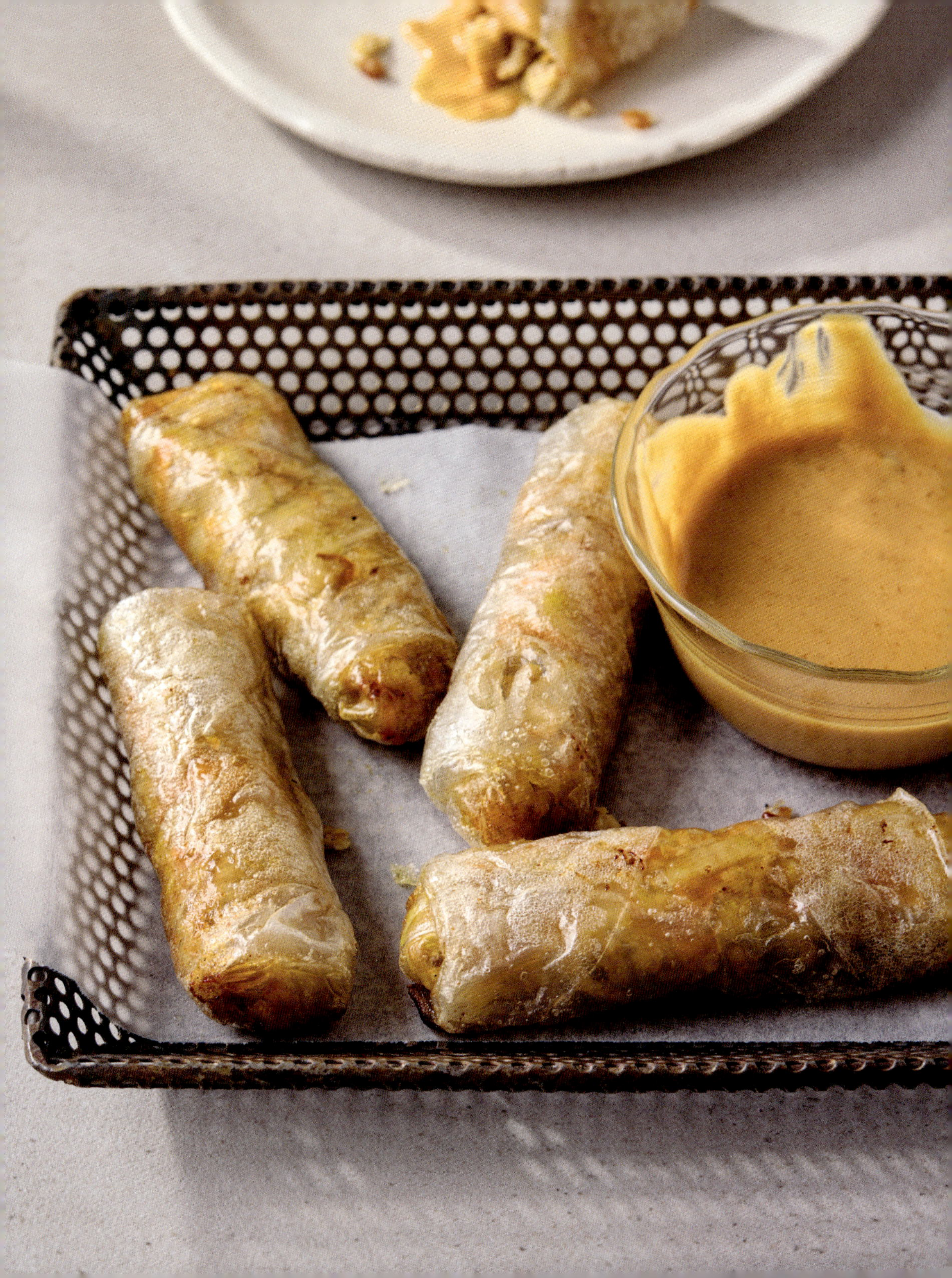

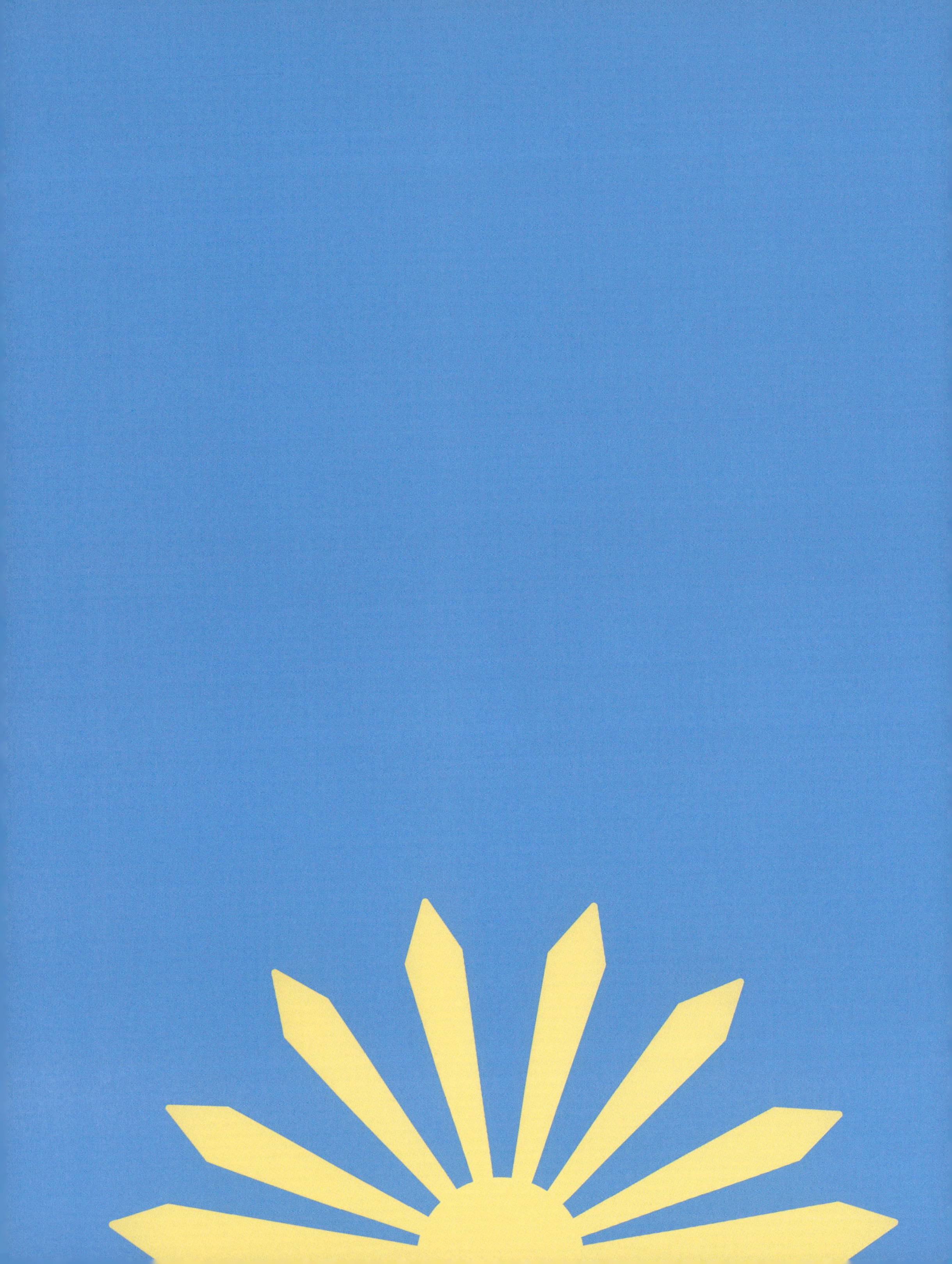

Snacks & Sweets

These tasty snacks and treats are ideal to keep stocked in the cupboard, fridge, or freezer, following the instructions in the recipe. From quick-boost energy balls that keep you going until dinner to delicious healthy desserts that always hit the spot when you fancy something sweet, you will turn to this chapter time and time again.

Crispy Sesame Tofu

Protein per serving: 25g **Kcals per serving: 359**

Serves 2

Prep + cook time: 35 minutes

- 280g (10oz) extra-firm tofu, patted dry and cut into 12 sticks
- 3 tbsp soy sauce
- 3 tbsp cornflour
- 2 tbsp plant-based milk
- 30g (¾ cup) panko breadcrumbs
- 1 tbsp mix of white and black sesame seeds
- vegetable or olive oil cooking spray

To serve:

sweet chilli sauce

1 Put the tofu into a baking dish, add the soy, and leave to marinate for 10 minutes.

2 Preheat the oven to 200°C (180°C fan/400°F/Gas 6).

3 Put the cornflour, milk, and panko into three separate shallow dishes. Add the sesame seeds to the panko dish and mix well.

4 Add a piece of tofu into the cornflour to coat, then transfer to the milk, and then to the panko. Place on a baking sheet and repeat with the remaining tofu.

5 Spray the tofu liberally with oil and cook for 20 minutes until crispy and golden in colour, then serve with sweet chilli sauce.

Keep it: These will keep in the freezer for up to 3 months.

Tofu is a complete plant protein and a source of calcium and iron, meaning this a snack that delivers more than just crunch.

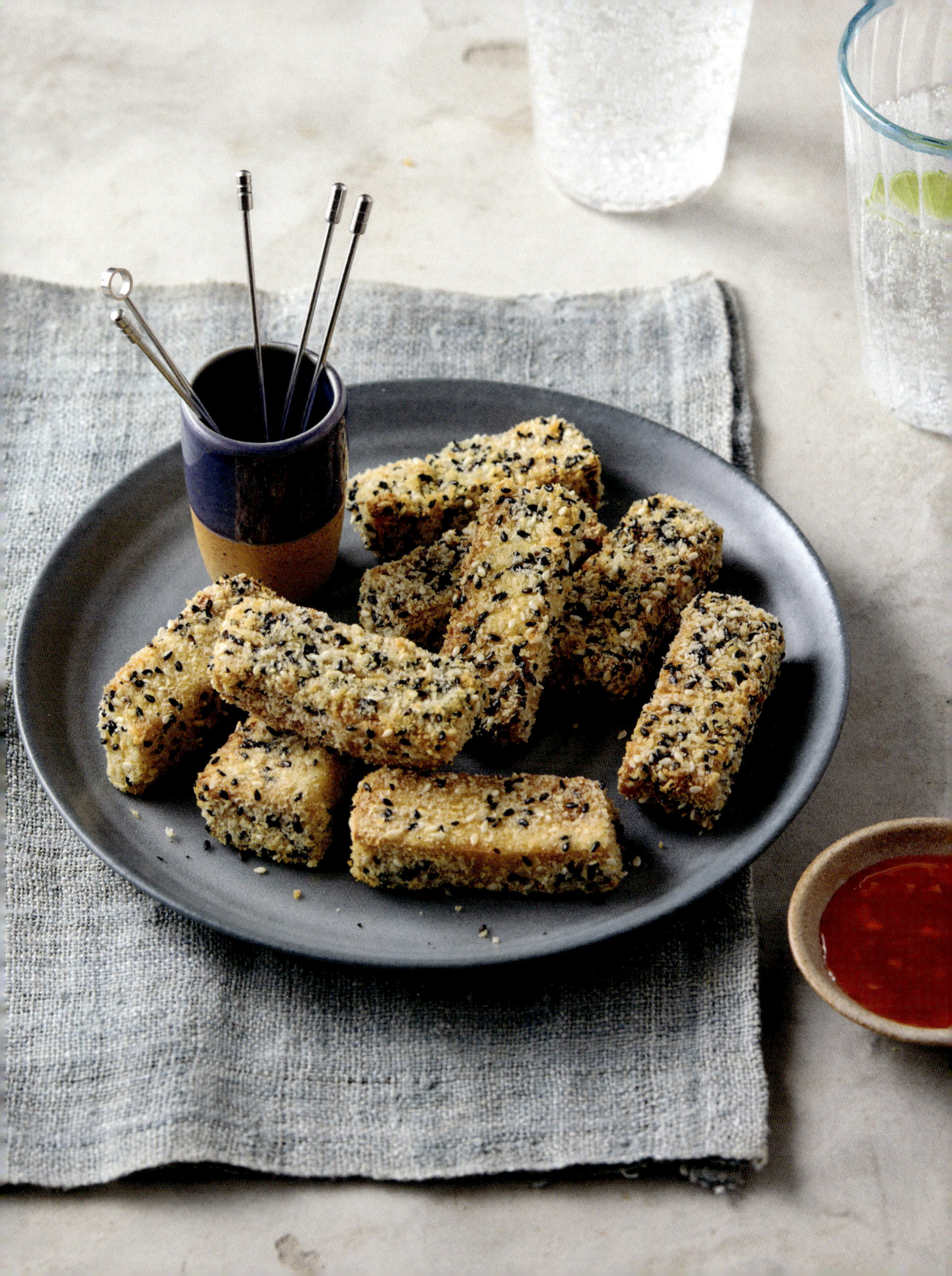

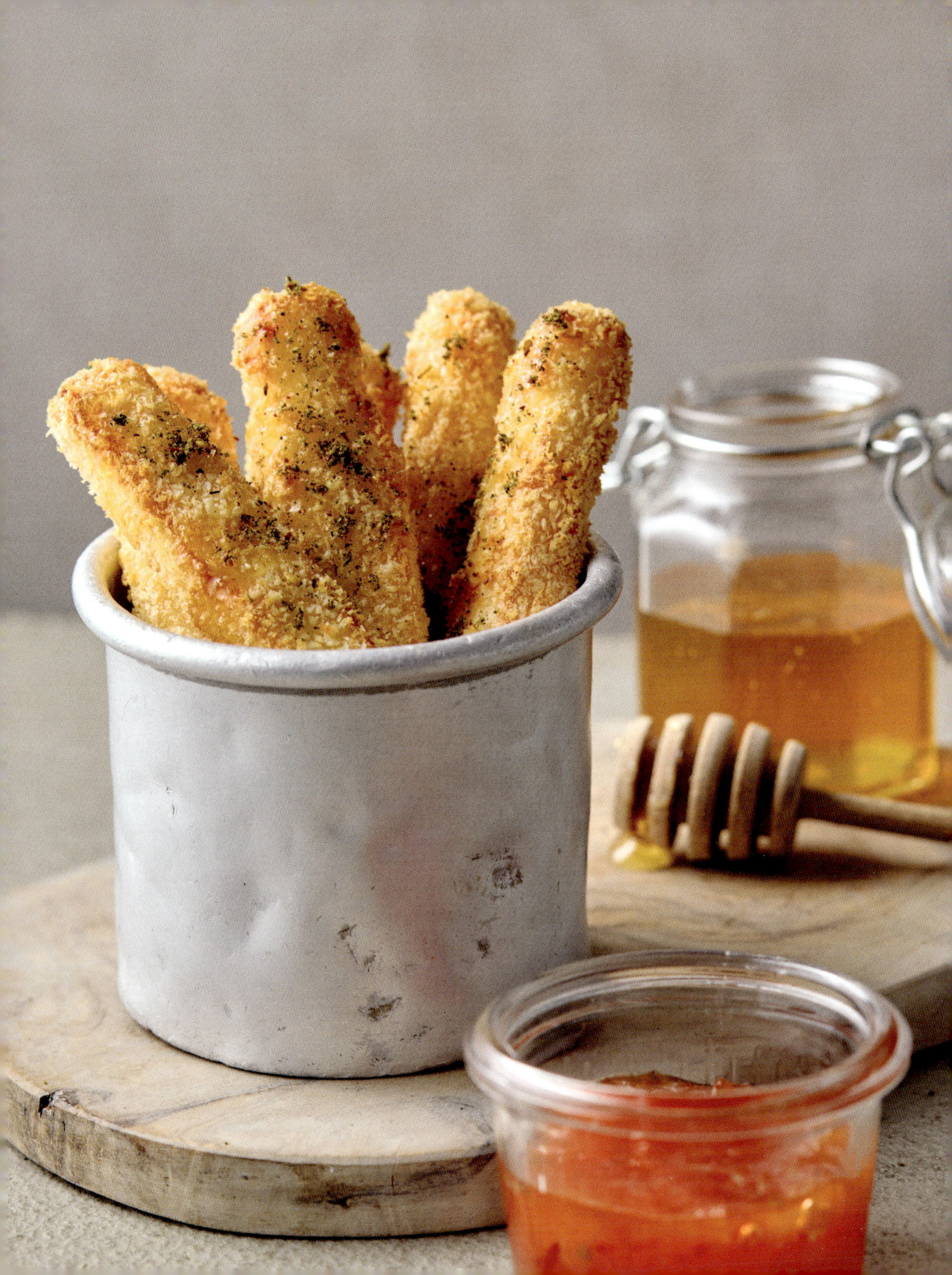

Halloumi Fries

Protein per serving: 34g **Kcals per serving: 535**

Serves 2

Prep + cook time: 20 minutes

1½ tbsp plain flour
1 large egg
50g (1¼ cup) panko breadcrumbs
1 tsp paprika
225g (8oz) pack of halloumi, cut in 2cm (¾in) batons
vegetable or olive oil cooking spray
salt

To serve (optional):
1 tbsp honey
1 tbsp za'atar
chilli jam

1 Preheat the oven to 200°C (180°C fan/ 400°F/Gas 6).

2 Put the flour, egg, and panko into three small shallow dishes. Whisk the egg well, add a pinch of salt to the flour, then add the paprika to the panko.

3 Put a halloumi baton into the flour, then the egg, then the panko. Put on a baking tray, and repeat this process with the rest of the halloumi.

4 Spray the halloumi bites generously with oil, then cook for 15 minutes until crisp and golden.

5 Serve on a platter, then drizzle over the honey, sprinkle over the za'atar, and serve with chilli jam.

Swap it: These would also work well with courgette.

Halloumi is a protein-rich cheese that provides calcium, making these fries a more satisfying, nutrient-dense snack than other fries.

Pea and Cottage Cheese Dip

Protein per serving: 12g **Kcals per serving: 363**

Serves 4

Prep + cook time: 15 minutes

- 1 bulb garlic
- 100ml (6½ tbsp) extra virgin olive oil
- 500g (scant 3¾ cups) frozen peas, defrosted
- 200g (scant 2 cups) cottage cheese
- 2 sprigs of mint, leaves picked
- grated zest of 1 lemon
- salt and freshly ground black pepper

1 Put the bulb of garlic in a small microwaveable bowl and add the olive oil. Cover and cook in the microwave on the lowest setting for 10 minutes until the garlic has softened. (Alternatively, peel the garlic cloves and put into a small saucepan along with the olive oil, and cook over a low heat until softened.) Set aside.

2 To a blender, add the peas, cottage cheese, mint, and lemon zest. Squeeze the garlic out of its skin into the blender, then season with salt and freshly ground black pepper. Blitz until combined.

3 Top with an extra pinch of freshly ground black pepper and serve.

Tip: If you are short of time, simply skip the garlic step and add in 2 tablespoons garlic and herb cream cheese.

Cottage cheese adds a creamy boost of complete protein, while peas bring extra plant-based protein and fibre to this smart snack with a fresh twist.

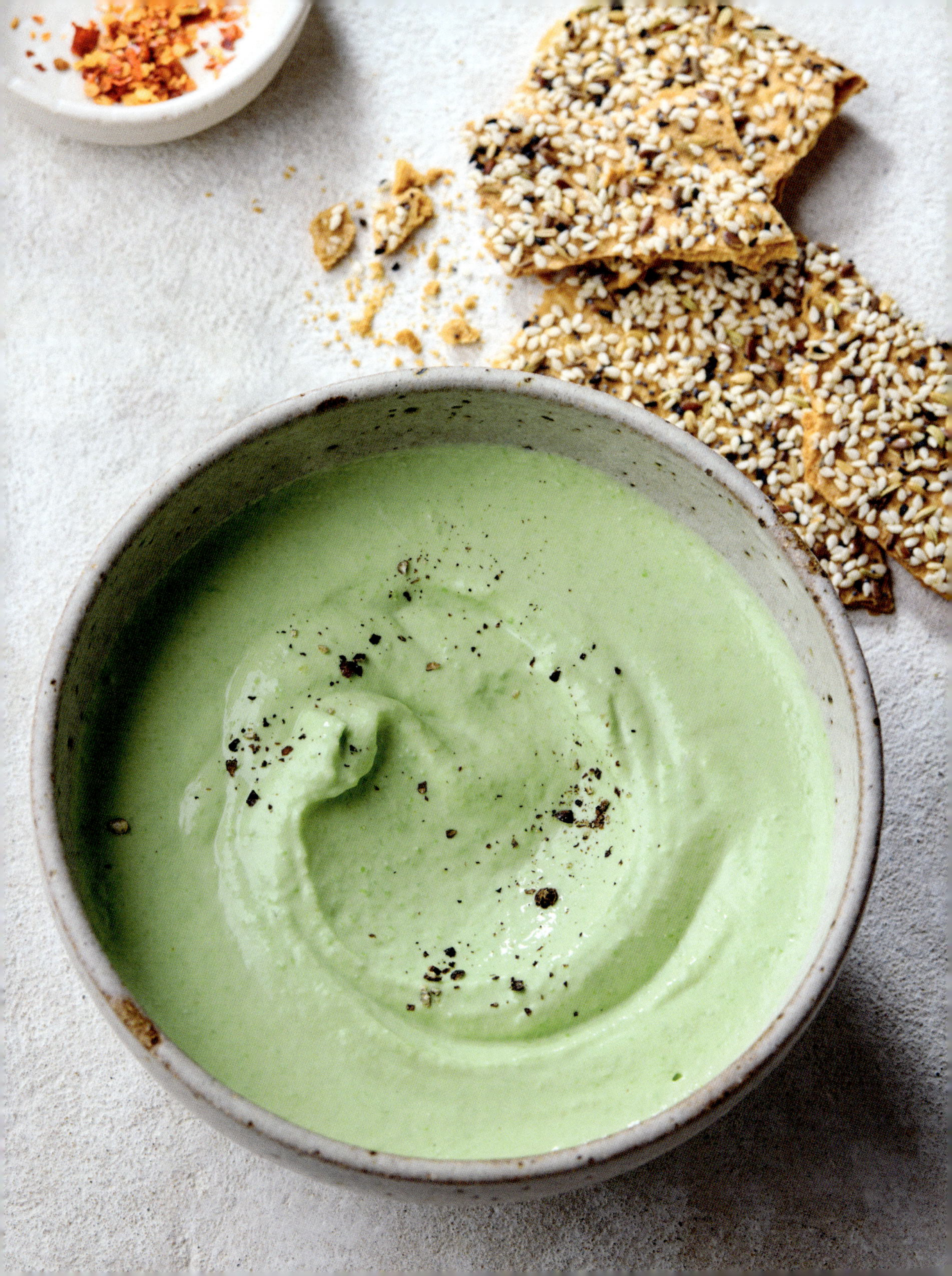

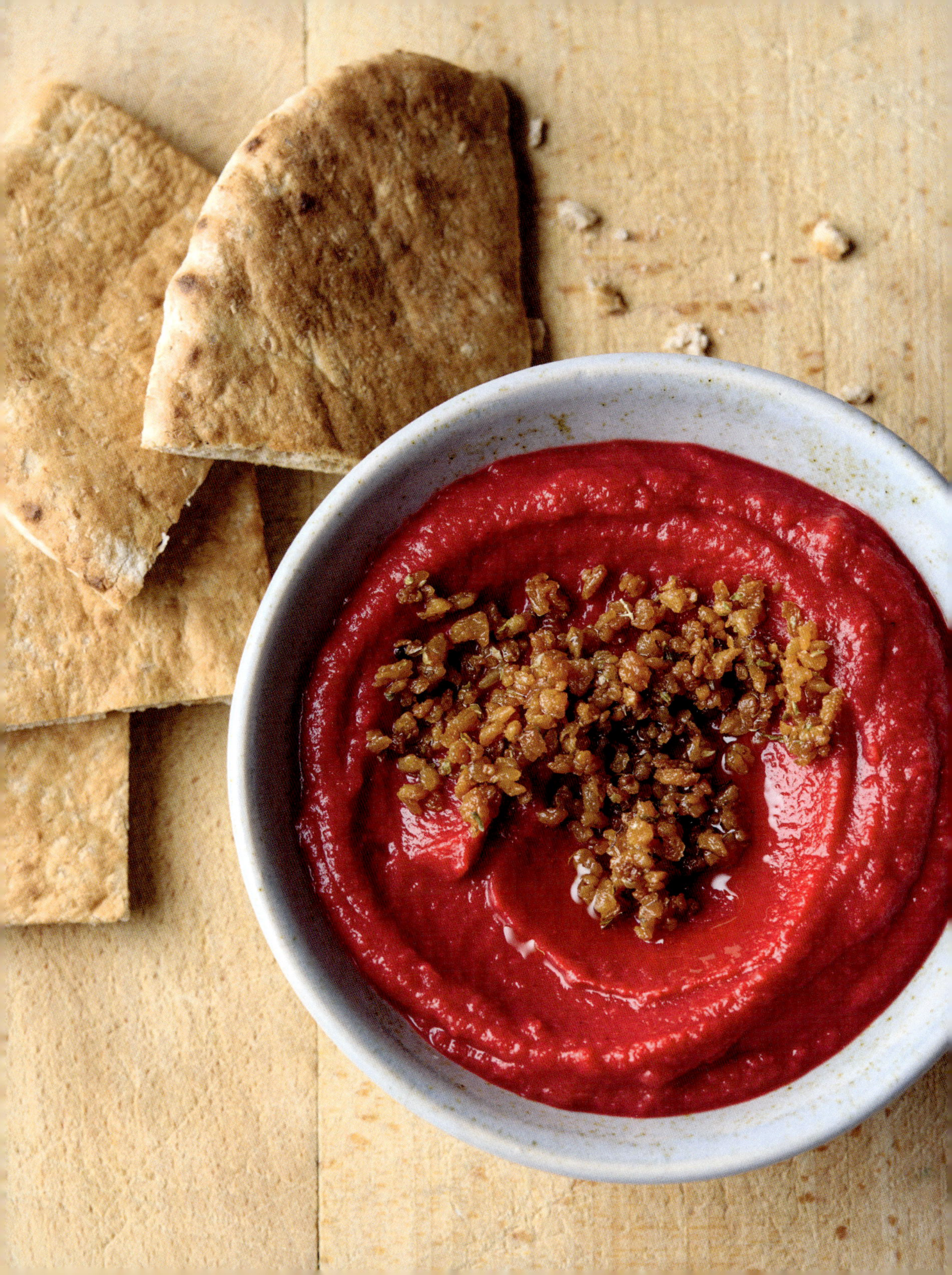

Beetroot Hummus

Protein per serving: 14g **Kcals per serving: 233**

Serves 4

Prep time: 15 minutes

- 1 tbsp bouillon powder
- 200ml (scant 1 cup) boiling water
- 50g (1¾oz) TVP
- 400g (14oz) can of butter beans, drained and rinsed
- 300g (10½oz) cooked beetroot
- ½ clove of garlic, roughly chopped
- juice of 1 lemon
- 1 tbsp extra virgin olive oil
- 1 tsp ground cumin
- 1 tsp dried oregano
- salt and freshly ground black pepper

1 Add the bouillon powder and boiling water toa measuring jug and stir well.

2 Put the TVP in a bowl and pour over the boiling stock. Let it sit for 3 minutes.

3 Drain the TVP out into a sieve, squeeze out the water with the back of a spoon, then set aside.

4 Meanwhile, to a blender, add the butter beans, beetroot, garlic, and lemon juice. Season with salt and freshly ground black pepper, blitz until smooth, then set aside.

5 Add the olive oil to a frying pan and set over a high heat. Add the TVP and fry until crispy and golden. Add the cumin, oregano, and a pinch of salt. Cook for 30 seconds more.

6 Serve the hummus topped with the TVP.

Tip: Leave out the TVP to keep this dip extra simple.

Packed with plant protein from butter beans and TVP, this hummus also offers fibre and slow-release carbs.

Strawberry Pudding Pots

Protein per serving: 9g **Kcals per serving: 224**

Serves 4

Prep time: 15 minutes, plus chilling

- 80g (⅔ cup) chia seeds
- 220g (8oz) strawberries
- 200ml (scant 1 cup) milk of choice
- 1 tsp vanilla extract
- 100g (scant ½ cup) Greek yogurt
- 50g (1¾oz) granola

1 Divide the chia seeds among four small glass pots or tumbler glasses, then set aside.

2 To a blender, add 200g (7oz) strawberries, the milk, and vanilla extract. Blitz until smooth, then divide this among the four glasses.

3 Mix well with the chia seeds, then put into the fridge for 1 hour to set.

4 Remove from the fridge, then top with the yogurt, granola, and remaining strawberries.

Swap it: Swap the strawberries for whatever fruit you like. Mango would also work well here.

Chia seeds and Greek yogurt bring protein, fibre, and healthy fats to this naturally sweet, satisfying dessert.

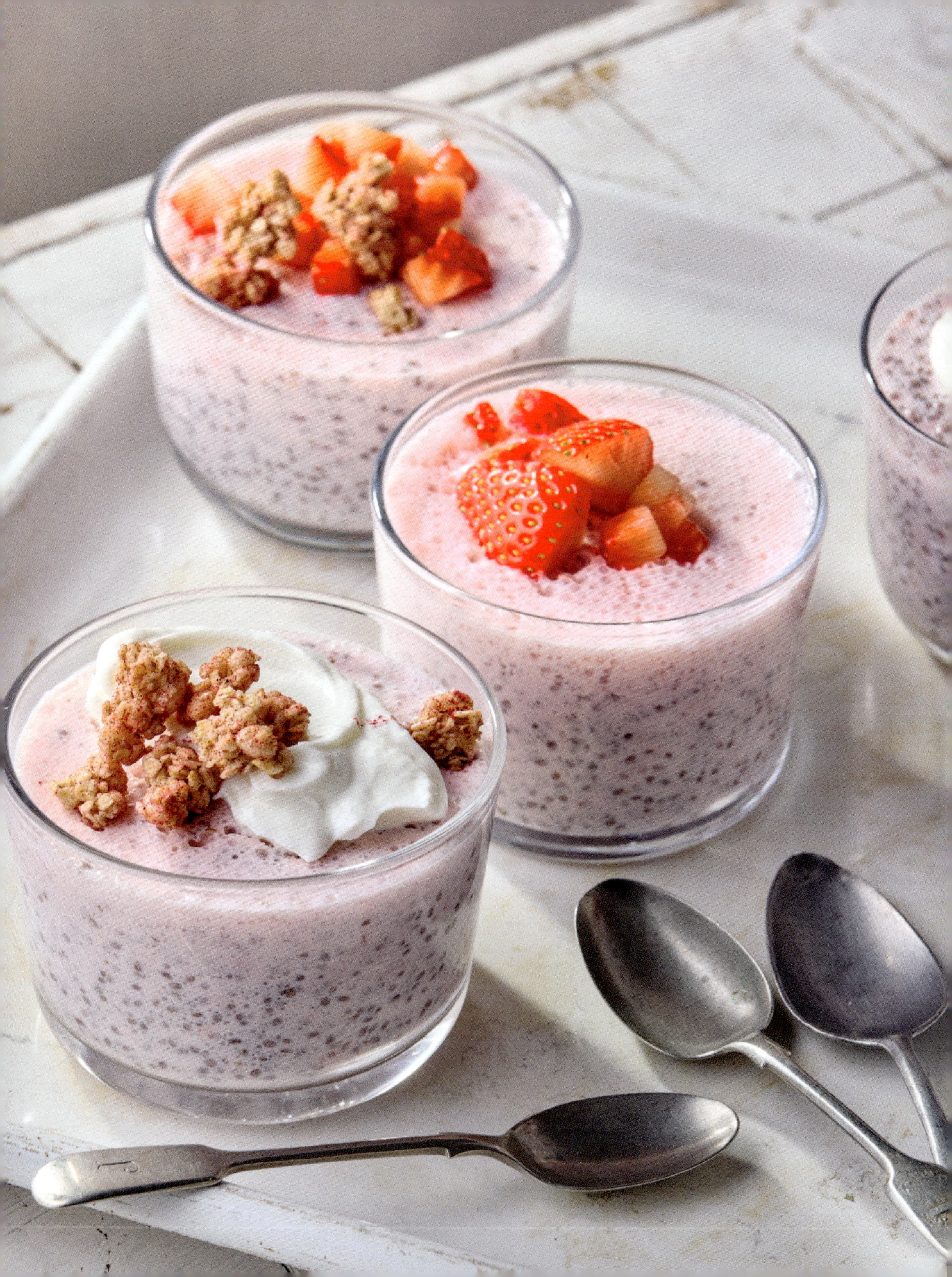

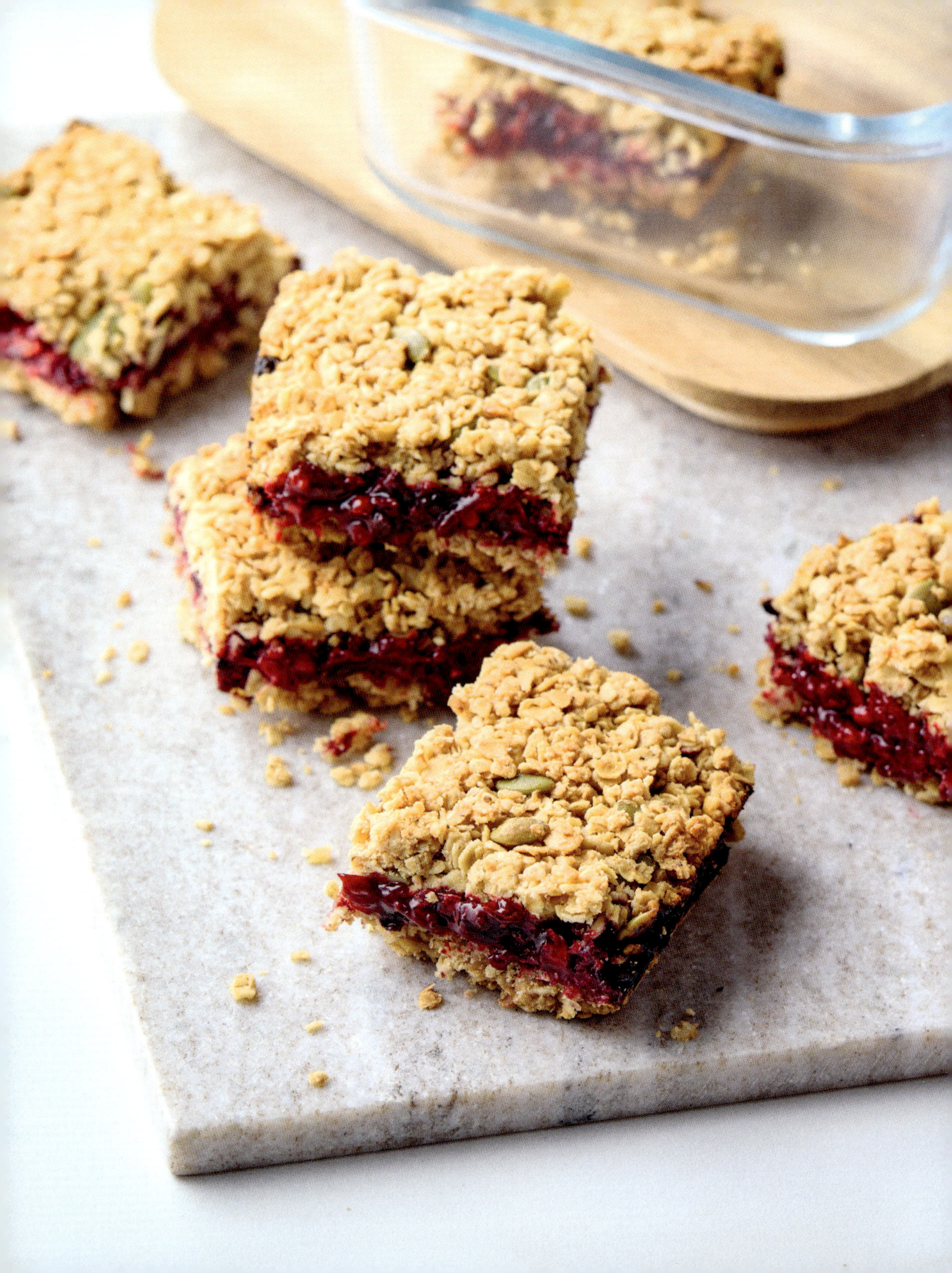

Protein Bars

Protein per serving: 10g **Kcals per serving: 327**

Serves 6

Prep + cook time: 35 minutes

- 200g (7oz) fresh or frozen mixed berries
- 200g (generous 2 cups) rolled porridge oats
- 30g (2 tbsp) coconut oil, melted, plus extra for greasing
- 100g (scant ½ cup) crunchy peanut butter
- 60ml (¼ cup) maple syrup
- 2 tbsp pumpkin seeds

1 Preheat the oven to 180°C (160°C fan/350°F/Gas 4). Grease and line a 900g (2lb) loaf tin, then set aside.

2 Put the berries in a saucepan, add a splash of water, and cook over a medium heat for a few minutes until they become soft and jammy. Set aside.

3 Meanwhile, combine the oats, coconut oil, peanut butter, maple syrup, and pumpkin seeds in a bowl. Mix well, then add half of the mixture to the prepared tin, pressing and smoothing the mixture down.

4 Spread the berry mixture over the top, making sure the oats are fully covered. Top with the remaining oats, pressing and smoothing down to cover the berry layer.

5 Bake for 25 minutes, then cool completely and cut into bars.

Keep it: Store in an airtight container for up to 4 days.

Peanut butter and pumpkin seeds provide plant-based protein and healthy fats, while oats and berries add fibre and natural sweetness.

Peanut Butter Energy Balls

Protein per ball: 3g **Kcals per ball: 94**

Makes 10

Prep time: 5 minutes, plus chilling

- 100g (1 cup) rolled porridge oats
- 2 tbsp crunchy peanut butter
- 40g (5 tbsp) flaxseeds or chia seeds
- 1 tbsp maple syrup
- 2 tbsp sesame seeds

1 Put all of the ingredients, except the sesame seeds, into a blender. Add 2 tablespoons water and blitz until the mix comes together and feels sticky in your hand. If needed, add more water, a little at a time.

2 Put the sesame seeds into a small bowl.

3 Roll the mix into 10 small balls, then drop them into the sesame seeds, pressing them down on all sides so that the seeds stick.

4 Line them up onto a baking tray and put them into the fridge for 20 minutes to firm up.

Keep it: Store in an airtight container in the fridge for up to 1 week, or freeze for 3 months.

Swap it: Try cashew or almond butter instead of peanut butter.

These no-bake bites combine plant protein, fibre, and healthy fats – a simple, energizing snack to help curb hunger and support steady energy.

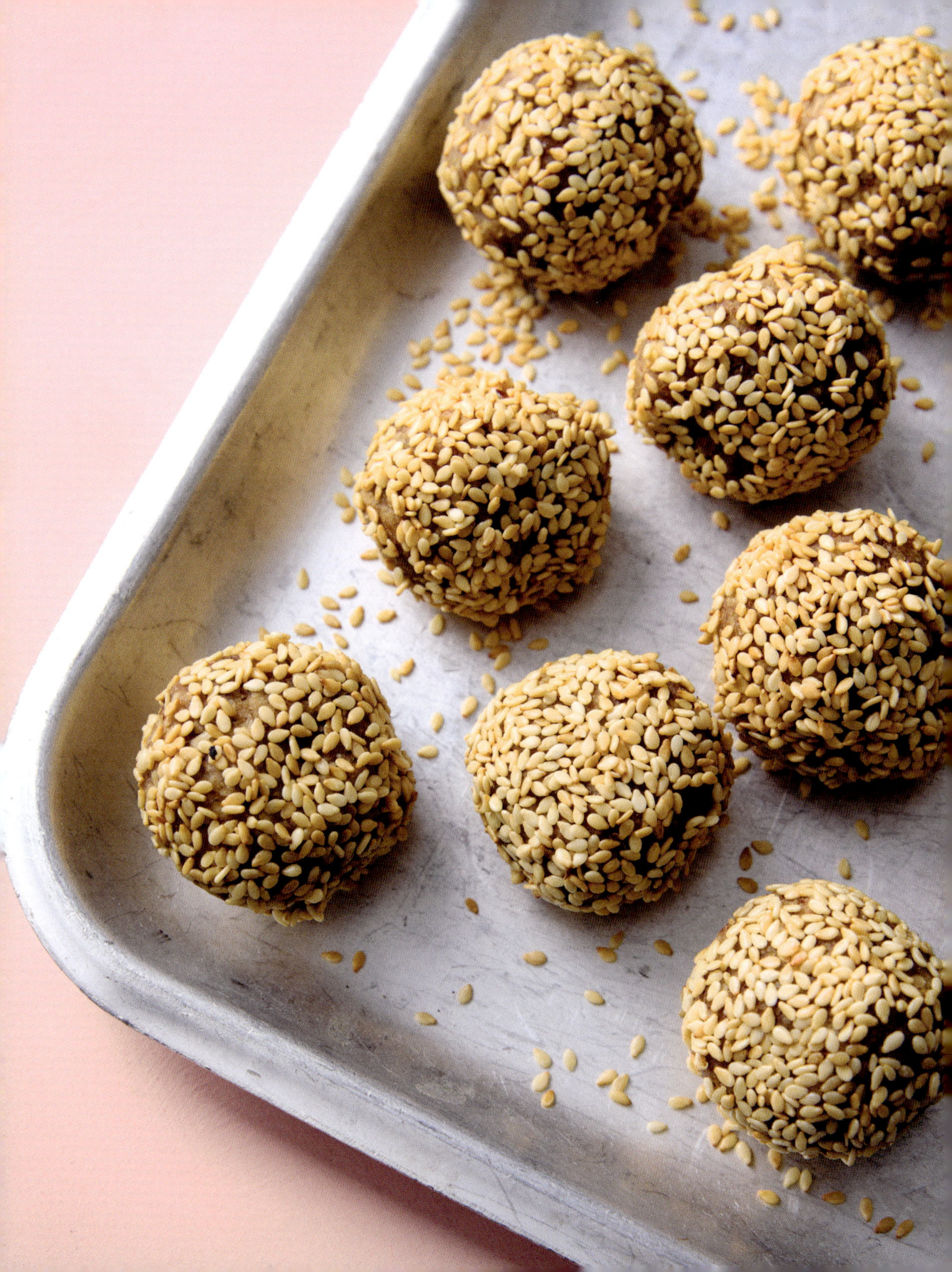

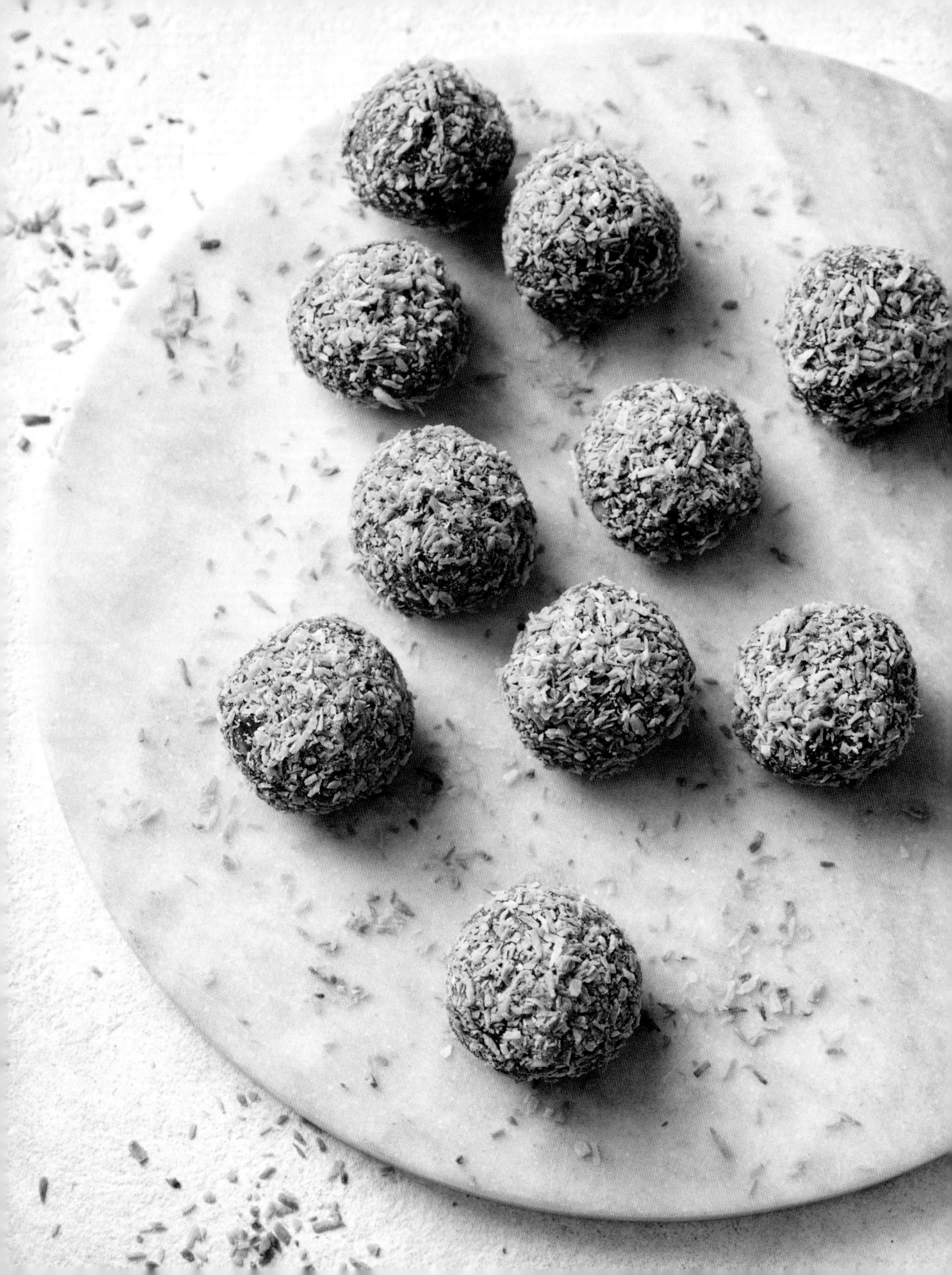

Date and Chocolate Energy Balls

Protein per ball: 3g **Kcals per ball: 119**

Makes 10

Prep time: 5 minutes, plus chilling

- 100g (1 cup) rolled porridge oats
- 2 tbsp cocoa powder
- 100g (¾ cup) pitted dates
- 50g (generous ⅓ cup) blanched almonds
- 3 tbsp desiccated coconut

These energy balls combine fibre-rich oats and dates with almonds for plant-based protein and healthy fats – a naturally sweet, nourishing snack to keep you going.

1 Put all of the ingredients, except for the desiccated coconut, into a blender. Add 2 tablespoons water and blitz until the mix comes together and feels sticky in your hand. If needed, add more water, a little at a time.

2 Put the desiccated coconut into a small bowl.

3 Roll the mix into 10 small balls, then drop them into the desiccated coconut, pressing them down on all sides so that the coconut sticks.

4 Line them up on a baking tray and put them into the fridge for 20 minutes to firm up.

Keep it: Store in an airtight container in the fridge for up to 1 week, or freeze for up to 3 months.

Tip: These are still tasty without the desiccated coconut.

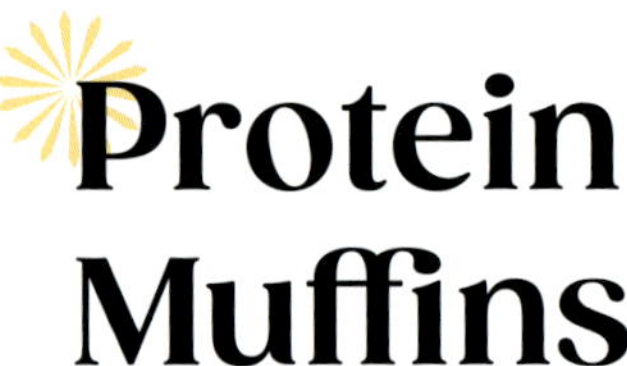

Protein Muffins

Protein per muffin: 7g **Kcals per muffin: 154**

Makes 12

Prep + cook time: 15 minutes

- 2 ripe bananas
- 80ml (⅓ cup) maple syrup
- 250g (scant 1¼ cups) Greek yogurt
- 4 large eggs
- 2 tsp baking powder
- 250g (scant 2 cups) self-raising flour
- 2 tbsp cocoa powder
- 2 tbsp sunflower seeds (optional)

1 Preheat the oven to 200°C (180°C fan/400°F/ Gas 6). Line a 12-hole muffin pan with paper cases.

2 In a bowl, mash the bananas with a fork. Add the maple syrup, Greek yogurt, and eggs. Mix well, then add the baking powder, self-raising flour, and cocoa powder. Mix well until combined.

3 Divide the mixture among the muffin cases and sprinkle the sunflower seeds on top, if using.

4 Bake for 12 minutes until a skewer comes out clean.

Keep it: These will freeze well for up to 3 months.

Made with Greek yogurt, these muffins get a natural protein boost and a soft texture, making them a smart way to add extra nourishment to your day.

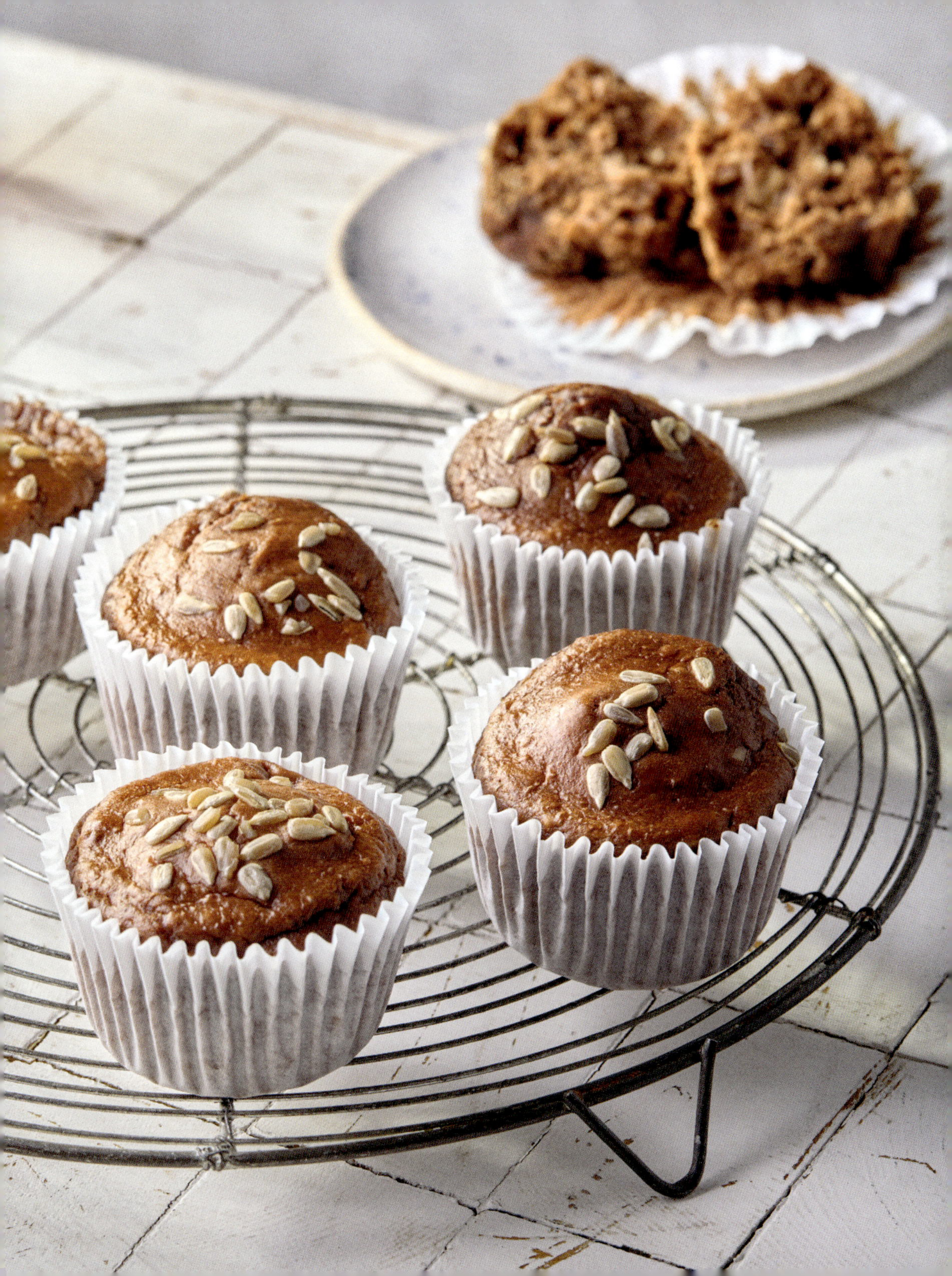

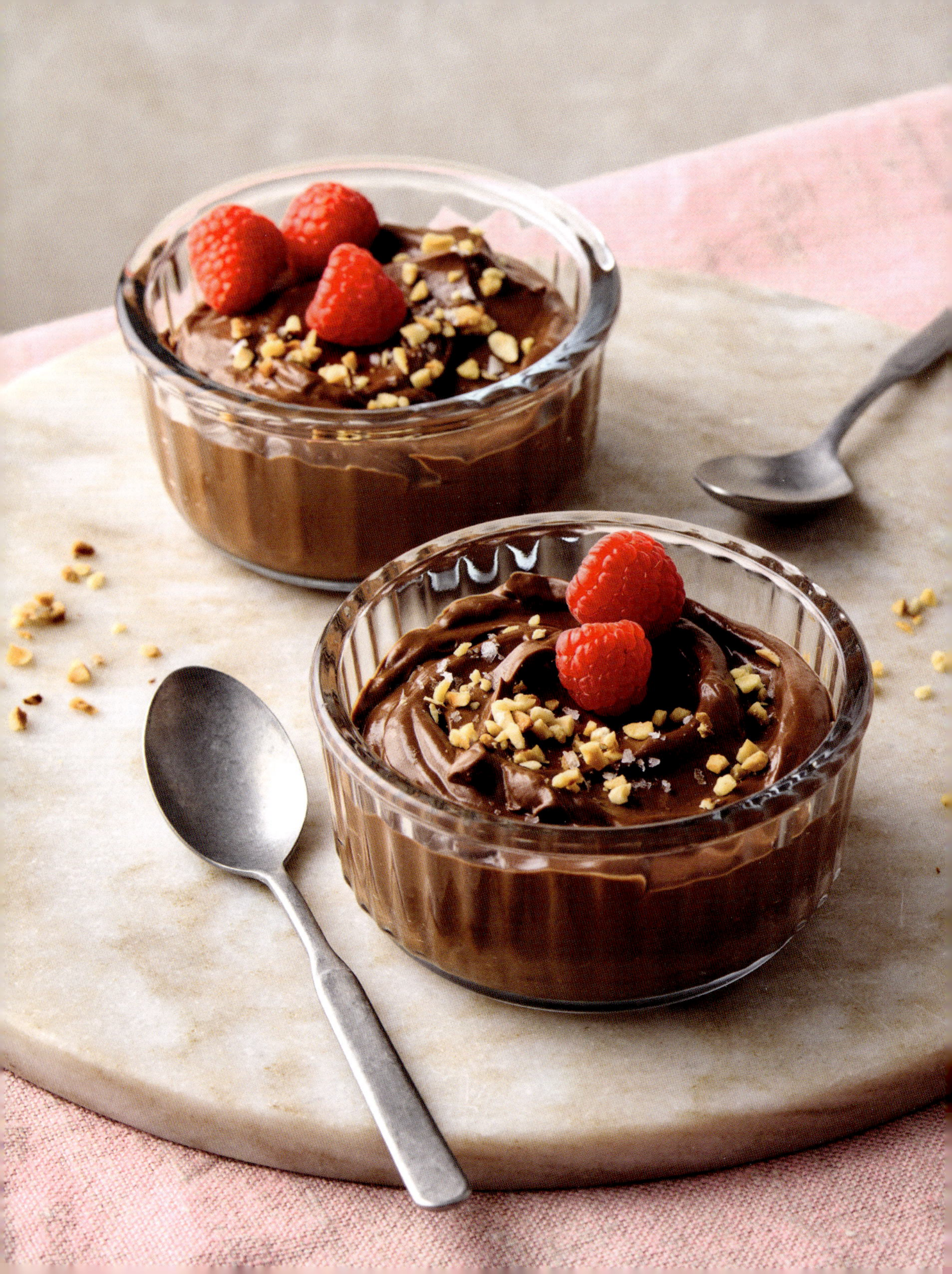

Chocolate Mousse

Protein per serving: 11g **Kcals per serving: 438**

Serves 3

Prep + cook time: 10 minutes, plus chilling

- 150g (5¼oz) dark chocolate, roughly chopped
- 300g (10½oz) silken tofu
- 2 tbsp maple syrup
- 3 tbsp roasted hazelnuts, roughly chopped

To serve (optional):

handful of raspberries

1 Fill a large saucepan halfway with water, and set over a low-medium heat.

2 Add the chocolate to a large heatproof bowl and set it over the saucepan, making sure the bowl is not touching the water. Melt the chocolate slowly, stirring regularly. Once melted, set aside to cool slightly.

3 Meanwhile, add the silken tofu and maple syrup to a blender, then blitz until smooth. Add to the bowl of melted chocolate, then fold together until fully combined.

4 Transfer to ramekins, and set in the fridge for 1 hour or overnight.

5 Top with the nuts and raspberries, if using, and serve.

Swap it: Swap the raspberries for any other fruits you may have. Bananas and strawberries work well here.

This rich, creamy mousse gets its protein boost from silken tofu – a plant-based twist that adds satisfying substance without compromising on indulgence.

Conversion Charts

MEASURES

North America, New Zealand, and the United Kingdom use a 5ml teaspoon and a 15ml tablespoon. North American measuring cups hold approximately 240ml. An Australian metric measuring cup holds approximately 250ml; one Australian metric tablespoon holds 20ml; one Australian metric teaspoon holds 5ml.

The difference between one country's measuring cups and another's is within a two- or three-teaspoon variance and will not affect your cooking results. All cup and spoon measurements are level.

The most accurate way of measuring dry ingredients is to weigh them.

When measuring liquids, use a clear glass or plastic jug with metric markings. We use extra-large eggs with an average weight of 60g each.

DRY MEASURES

metric	imperial
15g	½oz
30g	1oz
60g	2oz
90g	3oz
125g	4oz (¼lb)
155g	5oz
185g	6oz
220g	7oz
250g	8oz (½lb)
280g	9oz
315g	10oz
345g	11oz
375g	12oz (¾lb)
410g	13oz
440g	14oz
470g	15oz
500g	16oz (1lb)
750g	24oz (1½lb)
1kg	32oz (2lb)

LIQUID MEASURES

metric	imperial
30ml	1 fluid oz
60ml	2 fluid oz
100ml	3 fluid oz
125ml	4 fluid oz
150ml	5 fluid oz
190ml	6 fluid oz
250ml	8 fluid oz
300ml	10 fluid oz
500ml	16 fluid oz
600ml	20 fluid oz
1000ml (1 litre)	1¾ pints

LENGTH MEASURES

metric	imperial
3mm	⅛in
6mm	¼in
1cm	½in
2cm	¾in
2.5cm	1in
5cm	2in
6cm	2½in
8cm	3in
10cm	4in
13cm	5in
15cm	6in
18cm	7in
20cm	8in
22cm	9in
25cm	10in
28cm	11in
30cm	12in (1ft)

Index

A

almonds
date and chocolate energy balls **164**, 165
granola **42**, 43
apples: Bircher muesli **38,** 39
asparagus
smoked salmon and asparagus toast **26**, 27
spring salmon 88, **89**
aubergines
crispy aubergines with chickpea salad 134, **135**
slow cooker Thai green curry **118**, 119
avocados
blackened salmon bowl **144**, 145
breakfast tacos **34**, 35
chicken tacos **136**, 137
chipotle steak bowl 66, **67**
green lentil prawn salad 62, **63**
spicy tuna sushi bowl **60**, 61

B

bacon: chicken Caesar salad 130, **131**
bananas
mixed berry baked oats 32, **33**
porridge with nut butter 44, **45**
protein muffins 166, **167**
beans
beetroot hummus **156**, 157
breakfast tacos **34**, 35
chilli con carne **98**, 99
chipotle steak bowl 66, **67**
Greek bean salad **56**, 57
slow cooker beef stew with butter
bean mash **90**, 91
Tuscan-style soup 54, **55**
beef
chilli con carne **98**, 99
chipotle steak bowl 66, **67**
cottage pie 116, **117**
slow cooker beef stew with butter
bean mash **90**, 91
steak and kimchi with dipping sauce **102**, 103
steak with chimichurri and sweet potato fries **78**, 79
beef bone broth, slow cooker 126, **127**
beetroot hummus **156**, 157
berries
mixed berry baked oats 32, **33**
protein bars **160**, 161
Bircher muesli **38**, 39
black bean sauce: tempeh and mushroom stir fry **52**, 53
black beans
breakfast tacos **34**, 35
Greek bean salad **56**, 57
blackened salmon bowl **144**, 145
blueberry pancakes 24, **25**
Bolognese, TVP **124**, 125
brazil nuts: Bircher muesli **38**, 39
bread
chicken Caesar salad 130, **131**
prawn toast **140**, 141
seeded cottage cheese bread 112, **113**
smashed peas on toast 20, **21**
smoked salmon and asparagus toast **26**, 27
turkey burgers **94**, 95
Tuscan-style soup 54, **55**
breakfast tacos **34**, 35
broccoli
pad Thai 92, **93**
slow cooker Thai green curry **118**, 119
broth, slow cooker beef bone 126, **127**
buffalo chicken wings **132**, 133
burgers
halloumi burgers 142, **143**
turkey burgers **94**, 95
butter beans
beetroot hummus **156**, 157
Greek bean salad **56**, 57
slow cooker beef stew with butter
bean mash **90**, 91
butternut squash lasagne **106**, 107

C

cabbage
blackened salmon bowl **144**, 145
halloumi burgers 142, **143**
Caesar salad, chicken 130, **131**
cannellini beans: Tuscan-style soup 54, **55**
capers
salmon pasta with peas 76, **77**
spring salmon 88, **89**
carrots
pad Thai 92, **93**
slow cooker beef bone broth 126, **127**
slow cooker beef stew with butter
bean mash **90**, 91
Tuscan-style soup 54, **55**
cashews
cashew pesto pasta 122, **123**
nut and seed butter 28, **29**
cheese
butternut squash lasagne **106**, 107
chicken tacos **136**, 137
crispy aubergines with chickpea salad 134, **135**
English muffins with frittata **30**, 31
halloumi burgers 142, **143**
halloumi fries **152**, 153
halloumi with chickpeas and spinach **74**, 75
masala omelette **22**, 23
scrambled tofu 40, **41**
shakshuka 36, **37**
smashed peas on toast 20, **21**

turkey burgers **94**, 95
chia seeds
peanut butter energy balls 162, **163**
strawberry pudding pots 158, **159**
chicken
buffalo chicken wings **132**, 133
chicken Caesar salad 130, **131**
chicken orzo salad **82**, 83
chicken pesto pasta 58, **59**
chicken spring rolls 146, **147**
chicken tacos **136**, 137
ginger chicken congee 50, **51**
krapow 80, **81**
mango chutney chicken sandwich filling 108, **109**
miso chicken with smacked cucumber **48**, 49
slow cooker chicken and green lentil soup **86**, 87
slow cooker Thai green curry **118**, 119
chickpeas
cashew pesto pasta 122, **123**
chicken orzo salad **82**, 83
chicken pesto pasta 58, **59**
crispy aubergines with chickpea salad 134, **135**
halloumi with chickpeas and spinach **74**, 75
herby falafels 100, **101**
chilli con carne **98**, 99
chimichurri **78**, 79
Chinese leaf cabbage: chicken spring rolls 146, **147**
chipotle steak bowl 66, **67**
chocolate
chocolate mousse **168**, 169
date and chocolate energy balls **164**, 165
protein muffins 166, **167**
chorizo: breakfast tacos **34**, 35
coconut, desiccated: date and chocolate energy balls **164**, 165
coconut milk
curried lentil soup **110**, 111
Goan fish curry 84, **85**
slow cooker Thai green curry **118**, 119
cod
Goan fish curry 84, **85**
soy steamed cod **70**, 71
congee, ginger chicken 50, **51**
cottage cheese
blueberry pancakes 24, **25**
buffalo chicken wings **132**, 133
butternut squash lasagne **106**, 107
pea and cottage cheese dip 154, **155**
seeded cottage cheese bread 112, **113**
smoked salmon and asparagus toast **26**, 27
cottage pie 116, **117**
crispy aubergines with chickpea salad 134, **135**
crispy gochujang tempeh 138, **139**
crispy sesame tofu 150, **151**
cucumber
blackened salmon bowl **144**, 145
chicken orzo salad **82**, 83
crispy aubergines with chickpea salad 134, **135**
Greek bean salad **56**, 57
green lentil prawn salad 62, **63**
smacked cucumber **48**, 49
curry
curried lentil soup **110**, 111
Goan fish curry 84, **85**
masala omelette **22**, 23
slow cooker Thai green curry **118**, 119

D

date and chocolate energy balls **164**, 165
dips
beetroot hummus **156**, 157
dipping sauces **102**, 103, 146, **147**
pea and cottage cheese dip 154, **155**

E

eggs
blueberry pancakes 24, **25**
breakfast tacos **34**, 35
chicken Caesar salad 130, **131**
English muffins with frittata **30**, 31
krapow 80, **81**
masala omelette **22**, 23
salmon rice bowl **64**, 65
shakshuka 36, **37**
smoked salmon and asparagus toast **26**, 27
spicy tuna sushi bowl **60**, 61
tempeh and mushroom stir fry **52**, 53
energy balls
date and chocolate energy balls **164**, 165
peanut butter energy balls 162, **163**
English muffins with frittata **30**, 31
equipment 14

F

falafels, herby 100, **101**
fish
blackened salmon bowl **144**, 145
fishcakes **120**, 121
Goan fish curry 84, **85**
salmon pasta with peas 76, **77**
salmon rice bowl **64**, 65
smoked salmon and asparagus toast **26**, 27
soy steamed cod **70**, 71
spicy tuna sushi bowl **60**, 61
spring salmon 88, **89**
flaxseeds
nut and seed butter 28, **29**
peanut butter energy balls 162, **163**
seeded cottage cheese bread 112, **113**
fries
halloumi fries **152**, 153
sweet potato fries **78**, 79
frittata, English muffins with **30**, 31

G

ginger
ginger chicken congee 50, **51**
miso chicken with smacked cucumber **48**, 49
soy steamed cod **70**, 71

Goan fish curry 84, **85**
gochujang: crispy gochujang tempeh 138, **139**
grains: Greek bean salad **56**, 57
granola **42**, 43
strawberry pudding pots 158, **159**
Greek bean salad **56**, 57
green beans: krapow 80, **81**

H

halloumi
halloumi burgers 142, **143**
halloumi fries **152**, 153
halloumi with chickpeas and spinach **74**, 75
hazelnuts
Bircher muesli **38**, 39
chocolate mousse **168**, 169
herbs
chimichurri **78**, 79
herby falafels 100, **101**
hummus
beetroot hummus **156**, 157
herby falafels 100, **101**

K

kale: Tuscan-style soup 54, **55**
kidney beans
chilli con carne **98**, 99
chipotle steak bowl 66, **67**
kimchi: steak and kimchi with dipping sauce **102**, 103
krapow 80, **81**

L

larb, pork 114, **115**
lasagne, butternut squash **106**, 107
lemons
chicken pesto pasta 58, **59**
halloumi with chickpeas and spinach **74**, 75
salmon pasta with peas 76, **77**
lentils
butternut squash lasagne **106**, 107
cashew pesto pasta 122, **123**
curried lentil soup **110**, 111
green lentil prawn salad 62, **63**
red lentil soup 104, **105**
slow cooker chicken and green lentil soup **86**, 87
lettuce
chicken Caesar salad 130, **131**
chicken tacos **136**, 137
chipotle steak bowl 66, **67**
herby falafels 100, **101**
pork larb 114, **115**
turkey burgers **94**, 95
limes
chipotle steak bowl 66, **67**
pork larb 114, **115**
salmon rice bowl **64**, 65

M

mango: blackened salmon bowl **144**, 145
mango chutney chicken sandwich filling 108, **109**
mapo tofu 72, **73**
masala omelette **22**, 23
milk: porridge with nut butter 44, **45**
miso chicken with smacked cucumber **48**, 49
mousse, chocolate **168**, 169
muesli, Bircher **38**, 39
muffins, English: English muffins with frittata **30**, 31
muffins, protein 166, **167**
mushrooms
steak and kimchi with dipping sauce **102**, 103
tempeh and mushroom stir fry **52**, 53

N

noodles
pad Thai 92, **93**
slow cooker chicken and green lentil soup **86**, 87
tempeh and mushroom stir fry **52**, 53
nori: spicy tuna sushi bowl **60**, 61
nut butter
nut and seed butter 28, **29**
porridge with nut butter 44, **45**
nuts 14
granola **42**, 43
nut and seed butter 28, **29**

O

oats
Bircher muesli **38**, 39
blueberry pancakes 24, **25**
date and chocolate energy balls **164**, 165
granola **42**, 43
mixed berry baked oats 32, **33**
peanut butter energy balls 162, **163**
porridge with nut butter 44, **45**
protein bars **160**, 161
seeded cottage cheese bread 112, **113**
olives
chicken pesto pasta 58, **59**
Greek bean salad **56**, 57
spring salmon 88, **89**
omelette, masala **22**, 23
orzo: chicken orzo salad **82**, 83

P

pad Thai 92, **93**
pak choi
steak and kimchi with dipping sauce **102**, 103
tempeh and mushroom stir fry **52**, 53
pancakes, blueberry 24, **25**
pasta
butternut squash lasagne **106**, 107
cashew pesto pasta 122, **123**
chicken orzo salad **82**, 83
chicken pesto pasta 58, **59**
salmon pasta with peas 76, **77**
TVP Bolognese **124**, 125
peanut butter
peanut butter energy balls 162, **163**
protein bars **160**, 161
peanuts
pad Thai 92, **93**
pork larb 114, **115**
salmon rice bowl **64**, 65
peas
blackened salmon bowl **144**, 145

English muffins with frittata **30**, 31
fishcakes **120**, 121
pea and cottage cheese dip 154, **155**
salmon pasta with peas 76, **77**
smashed peas on toast 20, **21**
spicy tuna sushi bowl **60**, 61
spring salmon 88, **89**
peppers
chicken pesto pasta 58, **59**
chilli con carne **98**, 99
English muffins with frittata **30**, 31
shakshuka 36, **37**
pesto
cashew pesto pasta 122, **123**
chicken pesto pasta 58, **59**
pie, cottage 116, **117**
pistachios: granola **42**, 43
pomegranate seeds: crispy aubergines with chickpea salad 134, **135**
pork
mapo tofu 72, **73**
pork larb 114, **115**
porridge with nut butter 44, **45**
potatoes
cottage pie 116, **117**
fishcakes **120**, 121
spring salmon 88, **89**
prawns
green lentil prawn salad 62, **63**
prawn toast **140**, 141
protein
benefits of a higher-protein diet 12–13
definition of "high protein" 7
how much protein do you need 10
sources of protein 9
why protein matters 7
protein bars **160**, 161
protein muffins 166, **167**
pumpkin seeds
Bircher muesli **38**, 39
cashew pesto pasta 122, **123**
granola **42**, 43
nut and seed butter 28, **29**
protein bars **160**, 161
seeded cottage cheese bread 112, **113**

Q

quinoa: blackened salmon bowl **144**, 145

R

radishes
green lentil prawn salad 62, **63**
smashed peas on toast 20, **21**
spicy tuna sushi bowl **60**, 61
raisins: granola **42**, 43
rice
chilli con carne **98**, 99
ginger chicken congee 50, **51**
Goan fish curry 84, **85**
krapow 80, **81**
mapo tofu 72, **73**
miso chicken with smacked cucumber **48**, 49
salmon rice bowl **64**, 65
spicy tuna sushi bowl **60**, 61
rocket
cashew pesto pasta 122, **123**
chicken orzo salad **82**, 83
chicken pesto pasta 58, **59**

S

salads
chicken Caesar salad 130, **131**
chicken orzo salad **82**, 83
crispy aubergines with chickpea salad 134, **135**
Greek bean salad **56**, 57
green lentil prawn salad 62, **63**
salmon
blackened salmon bowl **144**, 145
fishcakes **120**, 121
salmon pasta with peas 76, **77**
salmon rice bowl **64**, 65
smoked salmon and asparagus toast **26**, 27
spring salmon 88, **89**
sandwich filling, mango chutney chicken 108, **109**
scrambled tofu 40, **41**
seeds 14
nut and seed butter 28, **29**
seeded cottage cheese bread 112, **113**
see also individual types of seed
sesame seeds
crispy sesame tofu 150, **151**
halloumi burgers 142, **143**
miso chicken with smacked cucumber **48**, 49
peanut butter energy balls 162, **163**
porridge with nut butter 44, **45**
prawn toast **140**, 141
shakshuka 36, **37**
slow cooker recipes
slow cooker beef bone broth 126, **127**
slow cooker beef stew with butter bean mash **90**, 91
slow cooker chicken and green lentil soup **86**, 87
slow cooker Thai green curry **118**, 119
smacked cucumber **48**, 49
smashed peas on toast 20, **21**
smoked salmon
salmon pasta with peas 76, **77**
smoked salmon and asparagus toast **26**, 27
soups
curried lentil soup **110**, 111
red lentil soup 104, **105**
slow cooker chicken and green lentil soup **86**, 87
Tuscan-style soup 54, **55**
see also broths
soy steamed cod **70**, 71
spicy tuna sushi bowl **60**, 61
spinach
butternut squash lasagne **106**, 107

green lentil prawn salad 62, **63**
halloumi with chickpeas and spinach **74**, 75
masala omelette **22**, 23
spring rolls, chicken 146, **147**
spring salmon 88, **89**
squash: butternut squash lasagne **106**, 107
stew, slow cooker beef **90**, 91
stir fry, tempeh and mushroom **52**, 53
strawberry pudding pots 158, **159**
sugar snap peas: chicken orzo salad **82**, 83
sunflower seeds
granola **42**, 43
seeded cottage cheese bread 112, **113**
sushi: spicy tuna sushi bowl **60**, 61
sweet potatoes
chipotle steak bowl 66, **67**
red lentil soup 104, **105**
sweet potato fries **78**, 79
sweetcorn
chipotle steak bowl 66, **67**
steak and kimchi with dipping sauce **102**, 103

T

tacos
breakfast tacos **34**, 35
chicken tacos **136**, 137
tempeh
crispy gochujang tempeh 138, **139**
tempeh and mushroom stir fry **52**, 53
Tenderstem broccoli
pad Thai 92, **93**
Thai green curry, slow cooker **118**, 119
tips and tricks 14
toast
smashed peas on toast 20, **21**
smoked salmon and asparagus toast **26**, 27
tofu
chocolate mousse **168**, 169
crispy sesame tofu 150, **151**
mapo tofu 72, **73**
pad Thai 92, **93**
scrambled tofu 40, **41**
tomatoes
breakfast tacos **34**, 35
chicken Caesar salad 130, **131**
chicken orzo salad **82**, 83
chicken tacos **136**, 137
chilli con carne **98**, 99
curried lentil soup **110**, 111
Goan fish curry 84, **85**
Greek bean salad **56**, 57
green lentil prawn salad 62, **63**
herby falafels 100, **101**
mango chutney chicken sandwich filling 108, **109**
masala omelette **22**, 23
salmon rice bowl **64**, 65
scrambled tofu 40, **41**
shakshuka 36, **37**
Tuscan-style soup 54, **55**
TVP Bolognese **124**, 125
tortilla wraps
breakfast tacos **34**, 35
chicken tacos **136**, 137
tuna
fishcakes **120**, 121
spicy tuna sushi bowl **60**, 61
turkey burgers **94**, 95
Tuscan-style soup 54, **55**
TVP Bolognese **124**, 125

W

walnuts: granola **42**, 43

Y

yogurt: strawberry pudding pots 158, **159**

About the authors

Susanna Unsworth is a chef, food stylist, and writer based in London. She trained at Leiths School of Food and Wine.

Laura Clark is a registered dietitian and nutrition consultant. You can find out more about Laura's work at themenopausedietitian.co.uk and on Instagram @menopause.dietitian.

Publisher's acknowledgments

DK would like to thank Laura Clark for nutritional consultancy, Susannah Cohen for assistance with food styling, Kathryn Glendenning for proofreading, Rajoshi Chakraborty for design support, Ashok Kumar for pre-production image editing, and Vanessa Bird for providing the index.

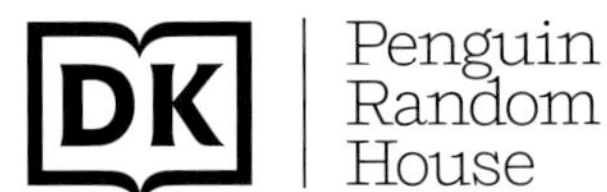

DK LONDON

Editorial Director Cara Armstrong
Senior Editor Lucy Sienkowska
Design Manager Tania Gomes
Senior Production Controller
Stephanie McConnell
DTP and Design Coordinator
Heather Blagden
Publishing Director
Stephanie Jackson
Art Director Maxine Pedliham

Author, Recipe Development, and Food Styling Susanna Unsworth
Design Abi Harshorne
Editorial Kate Reeves-Brown
Photography Tony Briscoe
Prop Styling Faye Wears

DK DELHI

Art Editor Devina Pagay
Senior Art Editor Ira Sharma
Project Editor Ankita Gupta
Managing Editor Saloni Singh
Managing Art Editor
Neha Ahuja Chowdhry
Pre-production designer
Satish Chandra Gaur
Pre-production and DTP Coordinator Pushpak Tyagi
Pre-production Manager
Balwant Singh
Production Manager Pankaj Sharma
Creative Head Malavika Talukder

First published in Great Britain in 2025 by
Dorling Kindersley Limited
20 Vauxhall Bridge Road,
London SW1V 2SA

The authorised representative in the EEA is
Dorling Kindersley Verlag GmbH. Arnulfstr. 124,
80636 Munich, Germany

10 9 8 7 6 5 4 3 2 1
001–356107–Sep/2025

A CIP catalogue record for this book is available from the British Library.
ISBN: 978-0-2417-8998-8

Printed and bound in Slovakia

www.dk.com

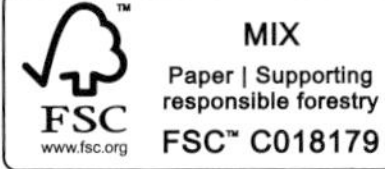

This book was made with Forest Stewardship Council™ certified paper – one small step in DK's commitment to a sustainable future.
Learn more at www.dk.com/uk/information/sustainability